Project Management in Health and Community Services

In the health and community service industries, projects are increasingly used as a way to develop new services and achieve change in existing ones. But in this complex environment, project managers need to be determined, flexible and prepared to respond to emerging evidence and stakeholder demands. *Project Management in Health and Community Services* challenges the accepted wisdom of project management methods from other fields, and presents new approaches to successfully implementing good ideas in health and community service agencies.

From the inception of a good idea, to convincing your supervisor to support your project, to wrapping up a successful outcome and capturing the lessons learnt, *Project Management in Health and Community Services* offers practical problem-solving strategies and a comprehensive guide to managing projects. It uses international case studies and examples from the field to illustrate a range of topics such as the project lifecycle, project planning, execution and evaluation, risk management, change, and effective teams.

Written by authors with years of practical experience and underpinned by recent research, this is a valuable resource for anyone studying or working in health and community services.

Project Management in Health and Community Services

Getting Good Ideas to Work

Judith Dwyer, Pauline Stanton and Valerie Thiessen

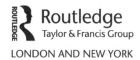

Routledge
Taylor & Francis Group

LONDON AND NEW YORK

First published 2004
by Routledge
11 New Fetter Lane, London EC4P 4EE, UK

Simultaneously published in the USA and Canada
by Routledge
29 West 35th Street, New York, NY 10001, USA

Simultaneously published in Australia and New Zealand
by Allen & Unwin
83 Alexander Street, Crows Nest, NSW 2065, Australia

Routledge is an imprint of the Taylor & Francis Group

Typeset in 10/11.5 pt Palatino by Midland Typesetters, Vic., Australia
Printed and bound in Singapore by South Wind Productions

British Library Cataloguing in Publication Data
A catalogue record for this book is available from the
British Library

Library of Congress Cataloging in Publication Data
A catalogue record for this book has been requested

ISBN 0-415-34052-7 (hbk)
ISBN 0-415-34053-5 (pbk)

To my mother, Joie Elwyn Dwyer, a born project manager. JD

To my sons Sean and Mark, my greatest projects. PS

To my father Peter and to Pamela, the thinker and the project manager. VT

CONTENTS

LIST OF FIGURES, TABLES

AND CASES

ABBREVIATIONS

CEO	Chief Executive Officer
CFT	Call for Tender
CPM	Critical Path Method
CQI	Continuous Quality Improvement
EOI	Expression of Interest
GP	General Practitioner
HRD	Human Resource Development
ICU	Intensive Care Unit
IP	Intellectual Property
IT	Information Technology
MET	Medical Emergency Team
MPHP	Municipal Public Health Plan
MRI	Magnetic Resonance Imaging
NDHP	National Demonstration Hospitals Program
PERT	Program Evaluation and Review Technique
PM	Project Management
PMBOK	Project Management Body of Knowledge
PMI	Project Management Institute
R&D	Research and Development
RFT	Request for Tender
WBS	Work Breakdown Structure

ABOUT THE AUTHORS

Associate Professor Judith Dwyer is the Head of the Department of Health Policy and Management at the La Trobe School of Public Health, where she teaches a Masters in Health Administration (in Melbourne and in China), and co-edits *Australian Health Review*, the premier national journal in health care management. Her research and consultancy work is focused on the governance of health systems and organisations. She was formerly a senior manager in the Australian health care system, and continues an active involvement in health policy debates. She received the inaugural AMA Women's Health Award for her sustained contribution to women's health care in Australia.

Dr Pauline Stanton is a Senior Lecturer in Management in the Graduate School of Management at La Trobe University, where she teaches in human resource management and employment relations in the MBA program. Her current research interests are human resource management in the health sector and human resource management effectiveness. She has previously worked in and with a variety of industries and organisations in the public and private sectors both in Australia and the UK. Her experience includes general management, project management, training and development and industrial relations. She has also travelled and taught extensively in China and has taken part in a number of research studies into different aspects of health service management. She has published a wide range of articles and papers and presented her research at a number of national and international conferences.

Since 1983, **Valerie Thiessen** has held a variety of hospital management positions including health information, casemix analysis, project and business management roles, in both the public and private sectors in Australia and the Middle East. Her experience also includes lecturing in health services management in the School of Public Health at La Trobe University, where she developed and implemented a web-based project management subject. More recently, Valerie has been involved in and consulted on a variety of projects including health information software development, patient information system implementation, and the development of education and training resources.

ACKNOWLEDGMENTS

We owe a large debt to the anonymous people who consented to be interviewed for the research for this book. We thank them for their generosity, honesty and insights into their own experiences of projects and project management, and their broader thinking about the discipline in the health and community services sector.

We are also grateful to several colleagues and friends who helped us with ideas, support, stories and resources, including Kathy Alexander, Anna Burgess, Alison Heywood, Terri Jackson, Libby Kalucy, Cynthia Langley, Sandra Leggat, Janny Maddern, Pete Middleton and Gregg Ryan, and the many colleagues who we have worked with and learnt from over the years.

Phrases and aphorisms used by the people we interviewed or from our own management language appear throughout this book. We have identified sources where we could, and ask forgiveness from those who invented the ones we couldn't identify.

INTRODUCTION

Like many good ideas, the idea for this book emerged during a conversation over coffee. The three of us were teaching project management to postgraduate students, mostly health service managers, in the School of Public Health at La Trobe University. During the conversation we complained that although there were many generalist reference books on project management there was little that captured the experience and addressed the needs of project managers in the health and community services sector. We began to talk about our own experience as project managers in a range of situations and realised that a book that drew on the richness of the industry and told the stories of the challenges, dilemmas and successes of the people within it had much to offer. We decided that we would write that book and base it around the experience of real people in a range of health and welfare organisations.

This good idea then had to go through the many stages of definition and redefinition, planning and implementation, always under pressure of time. Much more coffee was drunk and many stories told before the book was finally completed.

While we were writing, one of the authors was involved in a major building project—a house renovation—and we began many of our meetings with a progress report on her trials and tribulations, which seemed to mirror the difficulties project managers face with the people side of projects. This is her story:

When the builder didn't start on the agreed date we just shrugged and said 'that's builders for you'. After all, many people we know have had building work done and everyone has a building story, so a late start seemed par for the course. When he finally did get started six weeks later we breathed a sigh of relief and trusted that he knew what he was doing. When he disappeared for days on end on other jobs we thought 'that's builders for you'.

The completion date of 1 November became 30 November became Christmas and suddenly it was the end of January. I was working at home on the project management book. I had one eye on the book and one eye on the builder who appeared to be drowning in a sea of unfinished tasks. Eventually I could stand it no longer. I stamped outside, grabbed him by the collar and frog-marched him around the house pointing out all the unfinished tasks. Then, just as he was about to burst into tears, I sat him down at the kitchen table with a cup of coffee.

'Look Jim,' I said gently, 'you obviously have good building skills but not very good project management skills. I have good project management skills but poor building skills. How about we pool our skills and get this job knocked off in a few weeks—it will be a win–win situation—you get paid and we get our extension finished.'

'Oh yes,' he said, eyes brightening, 'what a good idea.'

So I looked at his little planning book—really a long list of unrelated and disorganised tasks. Taking a deep breath I said sweetly, 'How about we first of all set a goal—a finishing date—then we can rearrange these tasks into groupings or clusters, we can map out a plan of action and set timelines. Then we can break the job down week by week, day by day into manageable related tasks.'

The plan was perfect—it was all so logical and rational—it even had room for error and unforeseen events. I developed the week-by-week, day-by-day work schedule and set him to work. I boasted of my success to all and sundry.

But then came the control and monitoring phase. I did all the right things. I controlled, I monitored, I communicated, I facilitated, I negotiated, I cajoled, I threatened, I rang him up twice a day, I threw tantrums, I wrote him letters, I left notes pinned around the house—to his coffee cup, to his hat, to his tool box. I threatened to ring his wife. The work moved along in fits and starts.

One afternoon just when I was contemplating poisoning his coffee he came in and said, 'I want to thank you for all you have done these past few weeks—you have really kicked me up the arse and got me moving.'

'That's okay Jim,' I said through gritted teeth, 'as long as we get the job done.'

The new deadline came and went, another deadline was agreed and then another and another. I set my husband on him—even Mr Nice Guy has his limits. Then my sons joined in—if he disappeared off the job when I wasn't there, they would ring him and say, 'Mum's just been home—she was pretty angry to find you weren't here.'

He would scurry back and start working. Our combined efforts resulted in flurries of activity followed by a gradual slowdown. My dad came round to view progress—he took one look and sniffed, 'I've seen more work in a sick note.' The other tradesmen who came to do their work comforted and counselled me. 'You are doing a really good job,' they said. 'He was six months over on his last job—looks like it will only be four months over on this one—you're doing well.' That was no comfort for me, the project management princess.

But somehow my strategy of a good telling off, followed by a day in the doghouse, followed by sweetness and kindness, then back to the good telling off seemed to work. As far as I know, this strategy of punishment and reward does not appear in any of the project management texts as an implementation tool. Although you might find it in Machiavelli's *The Prince* or Sun Tzu's *The Art of War* (perhaps following the section on bringing discipline to unruly troops by beheading a few troublemakers).

However, as this book argues, flexibility is the key to project management success: there is no one way to make things happen and good ideas can be found anywhere. And if all else fails, remember Mao Zedong's four principles of guerilla war:

- the enemy advances, we retreat
- the enemy camps, we harass
- the enemy tires, we attack
- the enemy retreats, we pursue

and by the end of the book you should be able to manage any project—and even manage builders.

This story highlights the fact that managing people is often one of the most difficult parts of the project management process, a problem that is not limited to the health and community services industry; however, as a people-rich industry, it does hold particular challenges.

We were also increasingly aware that these early years of the twenty-first century are a critical time for health and community service organisations. While these organisations' potential to add to the quality and quantity of life of the people they serve has never been greater, that very potential has brought with it enormous pressure on resources. Old ways of funding, administering and managing health and social services were swept away in a great wave of change in the last two decades of the twentieth century, in both the rich and poor countries of the world.

Managers and professionals have responded with energy and creativity, finding new ways of providing care, and of doing business. Real sustained gains in effectiveness and productivity have been made. But at the same time, it has proven difficult to bring new methods into practice, to learn from research and to change old habits. The approach and methods of project management have a rich contribution to make as agencies continue to search for effective ways to innovate, change and grow.

This book seeks to address a growing need in the health and community services sector for concise and critical guidance in the use of projects: when to use the project approach, how to design projects for success and how to choose among the many methods and tools. The need is growing because more and more of what needs to be done in the sector is being conceived of, funded and managed as projects, while most of the literature on project management is designed for the engineering, IT or manufacturing industries. We aim to provide the information and the analytical framework that organisations, managers and project managers need in order to run successful projects, for the right outcomes, in a way which enhances the overarching purpose or strategy of their organisations.

Research for this book

Our research for this book included a review of the published project management literature, as well as reports of projects in the health and community services sector. We also conducted interviews with 13 senior managers in organisations representing a cross-section of the industry (large and small organisations, public and private, government and community). The interviews were taped, transcribed and analysed to enable us to form a picture of the major strategies, strengths, successes and problems with project management in this sector. We also collected project stories from champions, survivors and observers of projects from wherever we could find them.

While there is a wealth of published project management texts and resources, we found little that addresses the broad health and community services sector. For our purposes, this includes private and public agencies which provide health care and community services, and the government departments which administer funding, policy and infrastructure. While we have drawn primarily on Australian experience, we also bring perspectives from professional experience in the United Kingdom, China and Canada.

Using this book

We set out to write 'a critical and practical guide' to project management in health and community services. That is, we aim to provide readers with the analytical framework needed to understand and evaluate what is going on with projects in the field; and the means of choosing and using the right methods and tools for project success. The book has therefore been structured to meet a number of different requirements, for a range of audiences from students to CEOs.

The book is organised in two main parts. Part 1 explains the basics, provides a model for thinking about project success and failure, and addresses the context of the human services industry and its organisations. This part presents the big picture in project management and provides useful information about the factors that assist organisations to be successful in their project work. It will be useful as a background for the more practical material in the second part, and is aimed to meet the needs of senior managers who set the agenda for their organisations, including its project agenda. Part 1 is also essential reading for those who are new to the field (including students) and for those responsible for designing and administering programs which fund projects in human services.

In Part 2, the practice of project management is addressed, and the various methods, approaches and tools are reviewed, along with the challenge of making change happen through projects. We also provide a resource list of sources of further information and technical knowhow. Part 2 is designed to meet the needs of the practising project manager, and those entering the field of project management. It will be useful for those who plan, design, select, monitor and evaluate projects for their units or organisations, and for middle and senior managers who want to increase their success in getting projects approved and resourced. It is also essential reading for those who manage groups of projects, plan project strategy for their organisations, or lead the planning and development effort.

In the Conclusion, we aim to integrate the different perspectives, methods and issues covered through a consideration of organisational learning from the project experience and the need to ensure that project management doesn't become another fad.

We have included lots of headings and subheadings in each chapter to help the reader locate particular topics of interest, as well as understand the logical development of the material. A summary at the end of each chapter recaps the major points, and case studies and useful checklists are highlighted within the text for easy reference.

We hope that this book will be read by project managers, clinician managers, general managers, CEOs and the designers of funding programs, as well as students preparing for such roles. We welcome feedback from readers, and are still collecting project stories. We can be contacted at *project.stories@latrobe.edu.au.*

Part 1

PROJECTS, STRATEGY AND ORGANISATIONS

In Part 1 we define project mangement and explore its development in the challenging, often contested, ever-changing and people-rich environment of the health and community services sector. Part 1 aims to provide an analytical framework which will assist readers to make more effective use of the practical strategies that are presented in Part 2 for planning, designing and managing their projects.

In Chapter 1 we outline a framework for project management success which goes beyond the usual lists of 'critical success factors'. This framework recognises that characteristics of a project, such as planning and design, adequate resources and the performance of the project team, are influnced by underlying features in the health and community services sector and in each organisation.

In Chapter 2 we focus on these two underlying determinants of process success or failure: the sector and the organisation. The nature of the sector raises a number of challenges, including the seductions of project funding, the impact of idealism and managing the key stakeholders. Key features of the organisation include clear strategic directions, strong leadership and capable structures. We also explore building a project management culture and the people side of project management. Chapter 2 includes a brief discussion of managing projects in government departments.

Finally, we outline how this analysis might be used in practice, and we end the section with a discussion and a check-list featuring key questions intended to help practitioners choose good projects.

1

WHY PROJECT MANAGEMENT?

'Project management is turning a good idea into a successful outcome. You could have a great idea but if you don't have the skills to bring it to life in the real world it is only ever a good idea.' (*Experienced clinician manager*)

This chapter explains what projects are and what project management can deliver. It covers the origins and development of project management as a method, and the reasons for its increasing popularity. We briefly discuss what we have learnt about the way projects are used in health and community services, and introduce a framework for success in project management.

WHAT IS A PROJECT?

A project is an organised, time-limited, one-off effort towards a defined goal, which requires resources, and is traditionally described as having a '3D' objective (e.g. Rosenau 1998): to meet specifications, to finish on time and to do it within budget. In industries like building and construction, almost all production is structured into projects. Building a bridge is the archetypal example—you only build it once; you must complete the steps in the correct order, and bring the various materials, skills and resources together at the right times; there is a clear outcome; and there is always a deadline and a budget. To use an example closer to home, pharmaceutical companies typically use project management methods in the process of researching and developing new drugs, and in many ways the R&D divisions of pharmaceutical companies can be seen as simply a collection of projects.

Projects can vary in scope from something as simple as implementing the use of a new type of catheter to a complex undertaking like introducing a new model of care. Projects may be visible to the whole organisation and wider community, glamorous and exciting, or they may be hidden away in a small team or department—committed people doing good work.

Projects, programs and experts

In the health and community sectors there is a need to distinguish projects from programs. For a community health service, for example, developing and testing a Tai Chi program to enable older people to enhance their strength and balance is a project. Once the concept has been proven, the methods developed and the decision made to incorporate this approach, the regular offering of a 10-week Tai Chi program is not a project, but rather requires program management techniques to ensure that it remains effective and is delivered efficiently. While there is some overlap between program planning and design methods, and project management, there are some differences in that projects have a definite beginning and end whereas programs continue perhaps for many years and often evolve and develop. The term 'program management' is also used in the project management literature to mean 'a group of projects managed in a coordinated way' to obtain benefits not available from managing them individually (PMI 2000).

We also found that some people equate projects with the use of management consultants. Consultants are often used for projects, and the skills of managing consultants are an important aspect of project management capability in many organisations, but projects can be completed using entirely in-house staff and resources. The larger organisations we surveyed typically have some form of in-house project capability, people who play a role as project managers for the organisation and as internal consultants to support emerging project managers.

What is project management?

Project management is a set of methods and tools designed to enable organisations to plan, manage and achieve once-off tasks or goals. It sets out to solve the problems of defining what is needed, planning how to deliver it, managing the required resources in a timely and efficient manner, ensuring successful delivery and bedding down the outcomes.

Project management is increasingly used in all sorts of industries and organisations for several reasons, most of them to do with the pace and scope of change. In a world where new products and services are constantly replacing old standards, project management offers a method for driving the development process and whatever changes are needed for implementation. At the same time, products and services are becoming more complex. Many things that used to be able to be done by one person, or within one functional team, now require a broad range of knowledge and skill, as well as the resources of several parts of the organisation. The most typical example of this is the increasing need for any operational change in hospitals to involve not only the clinical or support unit which initiates the change, but also the information systems department.

Project management offers a different way of working together within an organisation, across departmental boundaries, to bring the necessary knowledge and resources to bear on a complex problem. This is particularly relevant to human services where changing the way people work together is often an explicit project goal.

In industry generally, relationships between organisations are also becoming more complex. For example, suppliers and contractors are increasingly working in alliances and partnerships with product makers and service providers. One of the main methods they use is conducting joint projects to develop and implement new ways of coordinating each party's contribution to 'the value chain'. Again, parallel developments can be seen in human services, in areas like child protection, mental health, emergency retrieval services and primary health care (Walker 2001). Multi-disciplinary teams are becoming more common in the sector, and the experience of working in an inter-disciplinary way is valuable preparation for project work.

As a result of all these trends, project management skills are needed by virtually all managers, as well as those who specialise in project management. Out of 236 respondents to a survey published in 2002 (White and Fortune), 63 per cent described themselves as managing the project, but not as project managers —they were managers, team leaders, senior managers, consultants and directors. This demonstrates the point that 'managers need to practise the skills of both general and project management, and the separation of the two areas of management is no longer necessary or desirable' (Healy 1997:2).

New problems, new solutions: the origins of modern project management

The capacity for innovation is a human characteristic, and major projects to achieve innovation have been completed throughout human history. Building the Great Wall, for example, or developing cities would have required some form of coordinated work towards a goal. But modern project management methods arose in the twentieth century.

There are two essential elements of modern project management. The first is a large set of tools and techniques for planning and coordinating the multiple inputs required for major projects. Henry Gantt, a pioneer in the field of scientific management, developed his famous chart (see Chapter 5) in the early twentieth century in a military context (Meredith and Mantel 2000) and perhaps he should be given the credit for the first project management tool. The 1950s saw the development of more advanced tools, including the Critical Path Method (developed by Du Pont to manage the shutdown of complex plants safely and efficiently) and the Program Evaluation and Review Technique (PERT), which was developed by the US military (Perce 1998).

The second key element is the role of the project manager and the project team. The defining characteristic of the project-manager role is that it has authority over the whole project, regardless of how many line management departments are involved. The first modern use of the project manager role occurred in the early 1950s, when Bechtel was appointed as the project manager for the Transmountain Oil Pipeline in Canada, and assigned one person to take overall responsibility for integrating the entire huge undertaking. At the same time, the US Air Force was beginning to use 'joint project offices' to integrate aircraft production projects (Stretton 1997). The need to find the right project manager and the right project team, people who understand and embrace this role and have the necessary skills to carry it out, has become a major factor in the development of the project management profession.

The emerging professional discipline of project management was subsequently developed, in the typical style of new professions, through the establishment of associations and other peak bodies (the 'clubs and societies' phase). The International Project Management Association (*www.ipma.ch*) was established in 1965 in Europe, the Project Management Institute (*www.pmi.org*) in the USA in 1969, and the Australian Institute of Project Management (*www.aipm.com.au*) in 1976 (Stretton 1997).

Project management, and the role of the project manager, spread rapidly throughout industry. The National Aeronautical and Space Agency became a major developer and user of project techniques from the 1960s, and improved on the '3D objective' statement with the slogan 'better, faster, cheaper' in the 1980s to describe their response to the need to work with tighter budgets. The information technology industry also adopted the practice of project management (for new product and service development) and provided the technology required for a proliferation of project management software, such as the popular Microsoft Project.

PROJECT MANAGEMENT APPROACHES

A survey of the methods actually used in project management in a range of public and private sector industries, conducted in the UK (White and Fortune 2002), found that in-house methods, developed and mandated by the respondents' organisations, were most popular, followed by basic tools such as Gantt charts and cost–benefit analysis.

The most popular criteria used by respondents for judging success were the standard 3D objectives (that is, being on time, on budget and meeting specifications). Other criteria included the fit between the project and the organisation and the results of the project for the organisation's performance—in terms of both business yield and minimising disruption caused by the project.

There is a wealth of literature which presents different approaches to project management. Perhaps the single most influential source is the Project Management Body of Knowledge (inevitably known as 'PMBOK'), published by the Project

7

Management Institute (Project Management Institute 2000). The PMBOK describes five key processes—initiating, planning, executing, controlling and closing—and nine key elements ('knowledge areas') in project management—scope management, time management, cost management, quality management, human resources management, communication, risk management, procurement (including contract) management and managing integration. We draw heavily on the PMBOK framework in this book and we have found that most project management approaches have significant commonalities with it. For example, Rosenau (1998) describes five key activities project definition, planning, leading, monitoring and completing.

Projects in health and community services

The use of project management methods is well established in the health and community services industries. Community services staff in local government, and in community health centres, began defining much of their community development and health promotion work as projects in the 1970s and 1980s, and developed in-house templates and protocols to plan and manage their work. These methods have proven effective, and are now standard practice in the community health and service areas.

Hospitals have been using project management methods for capital and IT projects for many years, but widespread application of these methods to their core business only began in the 1990s, learnt largely from management consultants and staff with community health backgrounds. The introduction of continuous quality improvement methods, and process re-engineering, were also important sources of project thinking and project skill development.

Australian health authorities, on the other hand, have tended to focus on the development of in-house approval processes and work flow management methods and, until recently, have been less systematic in adopting the key features of project management, other than in the capital and IT areas. Many central health authorities are skilled users of contracted projects, and it seems that there has often been a transfer of project skills from the consultants to departmental staff.

In human service organisations, project management methods are used for four basic purposes:

1. The development of new services, programs or technologies;
2. To improve existing services, care processes, work practices or service delivery models;
3. The implementation of new organisational structures or systems; and
4. The construction, installation and/or commissioning of new equipment and facilities.

Mainstream project management methods, with their origins in engineering, are best suited to the latter. Choosing, installing and commissioning a new MRI suite in a diagnostic centre, or building a new child care centre, for example, are tasks for which project management methods are ideal: they lend clarity, discipline and predictability to important decision-making, coordination and implementation tasks.

However, for the first three purposes listed above, the typical problems are fundamentally about the management of change and basic organisation strategy. The experience of Australian hospitals in projects to improve their 'bed management' (that is, the timely flow of patients into and out of an appropriate inpatient ward or unit) as part of the National Demonstration Hospitals Program is a good example. These projects set out to achieve change to longstanding work practices and relationships. While some of the difficulties were technical (for example, lack of a good automated information system), the more significant problems arose from fear of the consequences of loss of control of beds at clinical unit level, and failure to recognise the true scope of the task (Department of Health and Ageing 2002).

In Australian community services, projects are sometimes seen as a more participatory method of achieving change than traditional management decision making. The introduction of project initiation and approval processes in community health centres in the 1970s and 1980s was seen as a way of making both the use of resources and the processes of decision making more transparent and more amenable to shared decision making.

Is the sector getting value from projects?

Our research indicates that the use of projects is widespread throughout the industry, and that human service organisations of all types and sizes have established their own approaches to project management as part of their organisational strategy, with some impressive outcomes to show for their effort. However, we also found that while there is a lot of activity, many managers feel the results don't justify the effort, and project staff often end up frustrated when their work fails or simply 'fizzles out'.

The organisations we surveyed reported running anywhere from two to 80 major projects in a year, some with external funding, many initiated and resourced from within. Their projects included building and IT projects, developing new services and new service delivery models, quality improvement initiatives, policy development and research projects and re-developing or outsourcing support services. Organisational change was a constant underlying theme.

The larger organisations particularly reported difficulty in controlling their project agenda, for several reasons. They tended to overestimate what was achievable, and to lack discipline in the initiation and approval processes. One manager we interviewed expressed the view there were some 'quite deep-seated things that let this happen' and nominated lack of willingness by the leadership team to take on the task of imposing discipline, combined with government pressure to respond to its policy agenda, as important underlying causes.

PROJECT MANAGEMENT CHALLENGES IN HEALTH AND COMMUNITY SERVICES

The translation of management tools and techniques from industry generally to the human services sector is often difficult, requiring major alterations to suit the sector, and sometimes the promised benefits are never realised. Project management is just such an adopted method, and much of the literature does not adequately address the problems which arise in an industry so dominated by skilled professional labour, and so intimately linked to the processes and complexities of government and public policy.

Like any tool, project management can be well or badly suited to the chosen use, and can be well or badly used. Properly used, it has the potential to enhance the organisation's ability to innovate and grow; bring discipline to the processes of change; and enable organisations to focus more strongly on their purpose and the outcomes they need to achieve. In our attempt to provide insights into effective use of projects, we believed it was important to proceed from an understanding of the current realities of project management practice in the industry. We therefore turned first to an analysis of the typical problems encountered in project management in human services. We found several challenges which organisations need to meet in order to maximise their gains from the projects they conduct, described below.

The agenda: strategy or opportunism

Many human service organisations seem to find it particularly difficult to manage and predict their change agenda. They are often required to respond to government policies and initiatives in ways and at times decided by others. An increasing proportion of their total funding may be dependent on the submission of project plans in particular areas.

Human service agencies of all types often have mandates which require them to serve a broad range of patients/clients, and the resultant habit of thinking ('we must respond regardless') may spill over to their decision making about projects. Agencies might be keen to respond to their staff's good ideas and not miss out on new opportunities for funding or developing new services.

Whatever the reason, the organisations we surveyed all identified a problem in managing their project agenda. 'Doing 80 when we can only manage 20' was the way one senior manager put it. The large organisations in particular were busy, busy, busy but did not always have a clear picture of what they were actually doing and why they were doing it.

In the worst case, projects become a problem. Organisations distracted by project funding and project activity can lose focus on their strategic direction, with a resulting loss of coherence in their service offerings and operational strategies. Apart from the impact on core business, the projects themselves in this sort of environment often have little chance of delivering real benefits, and their results might be unsustainable when the project money is used up.

Contested ground: 'You want to change what?'

The purposes for which projects are used in human service agencies are dominated by the need to achieve change—change in work processes, change in service delivery patterns, change in professional roles and methods of working together, change

11

in organisational structures and reporting relationships, and the death and rebirth of organisations through amalgamations and mergers.

At the same time, there is a tendency in some organisations and professions to regard attention to organisational processes as 'soft' or a waste of time. There is cynicism arising from repeated waves of change and reorganisation, all of which have promised improvement while many have failed to deliver it, and which have in fact been dominated by the need to cut costs (Van Eyk et al. 2001).

Human service organisations are characterised by having multiple empowered stakeholders and being vulnerable to effective resistance by different groups. Various parts of the organisations may have very different goals, and operate under different and conflicting incentives. Projects flounder and some-times fail because they are trying to achieve things which are at odds with the culture, or which require unwelcome change in work practices, power relationships or ways of working together.

Project management methods have much to offer in the pursuit of effective innovation, and this potential is more likely to be realised if the size and scope of the change management component is recognised and planned for in the project design. In practice, project managers often find themselves devoting much of their time and energy to identifying, reporting and managing unforeseen (but predictable) conflict and resistance to the project. Project managers thus face the paradox that projects are seen as the way to achieve change, but often founder because the challenge of change is not adequately addressed in the design and planning phases.

Woolly thinking about worthy goals: hope is not a method

People working in human services are accustomed to living with complex goals which outstrip the ability of their organisations to deliver, and with the resultant unmet expectations of the community. For example, public hospitals typically aim to provide the broadest possible range of services, to the highest possible standard, for all comers. Patients, staff and the com-munity generally are distressed when, say, emergency services are not adequate to demand. But there is no ready solution to this problem, and it can be encountered regularly for years, with regular negative press as a result. Similarly, relatively small organisations dedicated to improving the health of particular community groups (for example, indigenous people, or children at risk, or people addicted to alcohol and other drugs) may make enormous contributions to the wellbeing of some members of their target group. At the same time the agency may not have any realistic hope of making a difference to the target group as a whole, or being seen by the public at large as having an impact.

The areas in which most health and community services agencies operate (even in the private sector) are subject to the vagaries of politics and public policy, one of which is the tendency not to acknowledge inherent tensions or conflicts in policy goals and service delivery methods. At the same time, staff are often strongly motivated by altruism, pride and a desire to achieve the best possible outcomes for their clients or patients, their organisations and themselves, whatever the odds.

These characteristics—the tendency to heroic effort and the acceptance of ambiguity and complexity—are necessary strengths. But they can be a problem in terms of effective delivery of projects. Projects depend on having, first of all, clear, agreed, achievable goals, and concrete 'deliverables'. In the human services environment, projects with worthy goals but with virtually no chance of delivering are sometimes commissioned. In the central offices of health and human service authorities, the sources of such woolly thinking can include the vagaries of responding to political agendas, the distance of the decision makers from practical realities and simple idealism. In hospitals and health services, problems of effective clinical governance (that is, the ability to make and implement decisions about the management of clinical services) can lead to the triumph of hope over practicality. Community-based organisations often suffer from a mismatch between the small size of their resources and their much larger goals.

Human service projects which straddle policy conflicts, or attempt to paper over unrealistic expectations, or go against the grain of important established practices and working relationships, are subject to false starts, delays and redefinitions. Sometimes, projects are used as a form of 'seduction', designed to convince policy makers and other key players to pursue a social policy goal by demonstrating how it can work in practice. This strategy can succeed, but issues like 'on time and on budget' are hardly relevant when 'specifications' are a moving target, or have many shapes in the eyes of several different stakeholders.

Our informants also identified problems like unclear and convoluted authorising processes, 'not enough spadework' at the beginning of projects, the power of charismatic people in the absence of due diligence, failure to allocate resources and basically poor project definition and planning.

Making it happen: skills, leadership and teamwork

The role of the skilled project manager was identified by all but two of the organisations we surveyed as a major determinant of project success or failure, and difficulties in establishing effective project teams were common themes in the interviews. These problems may be the result of resource constraints, of having too many projects and therefore spreading the project skills too thinly, or sometimes just from choosing 'the wrong project manager'.

The leadership challenge in project management occurs at two levels: the authorising level and the project team. Leadership is a disseminated role in human service organisations—sometimes because of a commitment to democratic and participative values, and sometimes because of the relative power and autonomy of large groups of professional staff. As is often the case in organisations with such defining characteristics, disseminated leadership is both a strength and a weakness for project management in human service organisations. On the one hand, it enables small-scale innovation; on the other, it can make whole-of-organisation change very difficult.

Because project managers must often acquire access to (or even temporary control of) resources which are the responsibility of functional managers and departments, there can be a problem in determining who has the authority to make decisions about issues on which the project's success depends. There is also a problem with conflicting loyalties among those staff who are temporarily seconded to a project—commitment to the project and the project team on the one hand, and to their ongoing functional group on the other. Good project outcomes depend on good project management, and on organisations successfully managing these potential conflicts.

Knowing how: tools, techniques and methods

As noted earlier in this chapter, the project management methods and tools currently available were designed, by and large, for engineering, manufacturing and IT projects, and while some of them are very adaptable, there are two key problems for their use in health and community services.

First, they tend to pay inadequate attention to the complexities of multiple stakeholders, multiple agendas and the politics of change that so often underlie project failure in the human services sector. In this situation the best project management skills might be good people skills such as communication and negotiation rather than adherence to a particular method.

Second, while most projects in the sector are fundamentally aimed at achieving change, the methods themselves can be quite rigid, mechanistic and bureaucratic—'death by process', as one CEO described it. This assessment is backed up by outcomes of the White and Fortune survey (2002), which included a finding that many of the tools and techniques were poor at modelling real-world problems.

Sometimes the method problem is even more basic: organisations may fail to recognise that they need a method, or may fail to identify that the activity they have embarked upon is a project, which needs to be managed.

Sustainability: did we get there?

When a project is designed and funded to change the way services are delivered, or to test a method for delivering a new service, there is often a fundamental assumption that if the new method works, it can be made to do so within existing resources. This assumption is often correct in that it may bring benefits, and cost reductions, at the somewhat theoretical level of 'the system' or 'the community'. But it is common experience that the costs are incurred by those who develop the new method and the savings accrue elsewhere. (The opposite is of course also true—that the innovator displaces costs onto other parts of the care system.)

The outcomes of projects might also prove difficult to sustain when the new methods have not really 'taken', or when those who stood to lose from the change are able to regroup and reclaim the old ways. This is particularly true if little thought has been given to how results might be integrated, or to what level of resources and support will be needed to sustain them.

Another important question for organisations is developing and sustaining their project capacity—keeping their good project managers, and embedding the skills of project management as part of their organisational knowledge. This aspect of organisation development is often overlooked or is not seen as a priority when it has to compete with other more essential areas of service delivery.

Is it the sector or is it the method?

We've outlined six challenges that the sector needs to address to get the maximum value from its use of the project approach. The alternative explanation needs to be considered: are these issues indicators of weaknesses in the method rather than of problems in the sector?

In a sense, projects are simply hived-off segments of the ongoing, complicated and messy business of the organisation in which they sit, with an artificial line drawn around them and some special rules and resources applied. The theoretical model of the project gives it a clear, uncontested goal, a set of technical requirements which can be fulfilled to meet the goal, and a set of methods and tools for doing so. The results are then handed back to grateful operating units that use them to move forward to a brighter, more effective and more competitive future. In recent years, the project management field has been claiming ever broader territory—for example, that whole organisations should be structured as groups of projects, with resultant gains in flexibility and speed of response to change (e.g. McElroy 1996).

However, it is argued that the growing use of projects is causing new problems. Managers don't know how to operate in environments that require more openness and more enduring commitment to a fixed goal, and are by and large not in favour of reducing their own discretion or power (Partington 1996). Public sector organisations work with complex goals and contested structures, policies and methods. Internal projects must deal with stakeholders who are in effect both the subjects and the objects of change—that is, the change makers and the changed. Thus, the project team may need to change the roles, mindsets or privileges of the very people who must endorse the project's goals and outcomes.

Projects bring their own bureaucracy and, paradoxically, are resistant to change in the project itself while advocating the use of projects to pursue organisational change. Finally, the methods of project management are not built on an adequate research and theory base, and cannot justify their claims to universal application.

This book is our answer to the question that started this section—that is, whether the method is sufficiently robust to serve the needs of the health and community services sector. And the answer is 'yes, for the right purposes and with modifications'. The rest of this book outlines how and why.

DEFINING PROJECT SUCCESS

It is not difficult to highlight the challenges and difficulties that health and community service organisations face in their project management practice, and many agencies are able to meet these challenges and develop and implement successful projects with sustainable outcomes. So as well as an overview of the typical difficulties human service organisations encounter with projects, we also needed a framework for analysing the sources of success and failure, and a clear understanding of what project success is.

Early studies of project management tended to focus on reasons for project failure rather than project success. Basically, if a project did not meet one of the 3Ds—on time, within budget and meeting the aims of the client—it was a failure (Belassi and Tukel 1996).

In reality the picture is much more complex and many projects go over time and budget, particularly in the human services area, but are still judged to be successful by participants for a variety of other reasons. In White and Fortune's 2002 survey of project managers across a range of industries, 41 per cent of them claimed complete success in the implementation of their projects (although this figure may overstate success rates in general because of the low 24 per cent response rate to this survey). White and Fortune compared the respondents' criteria for judging success against those reported in the literature and found that although the three most frequently cited criteria were the same (meeting clients' requirements, time taken and cost), other factors were also considered important. These factors included the fit between the project and the organisation (the extent to which the project met organisational objectives), and the consequences of the project for the performance of the business (for example, minimising business disruption as well as the project's yield in terms of business and other benefits). In other words the respondents judged the project's success or failure in a wider organisational context.

The environmental context also needs to be considered, as the researchers found that projects often had unexpected side-effects, 70 per cent of which could be attributed to lack of awareness of the environment. White and Fortune suggest that in many of the methods used, 'insufficient account was taken of project boundaries and environments' (2002:5).

Some of these side-effects were beneficial to the organis-ation—for example, an increase in business, sales or opportunities, or gaining new knowledge and understanding. Other benefits included improving business or staff relations and achieving greater consistency of work methods. Not all unexpected side-effects were beneficial, however. The undesirable effects were wide ranging and included organisational conflicts and problems with staff, clients, contractors and/or suppliers as well as technical limitations. Lack of awareness of the environment featured strongly here, as did the usual problems of under-estimating time and cost. Other problems included changes to goals and objectives, poor IT awareness or knowledge and conflicting priorities.

The other important variable in defining success is the question of stakeholders. In human services particularly, success must be judged from several perspectives—what clients or patients see as successful project outcomes might be very different from the views of owners or funders.

Determinants of success

Several authors have defined the factors critical to project success in different industries (e.g. Jang and Lee 1998; Zimmer 1999a). White and Fortune (2002) asked their respondents to rank the three critical success factors for their projects. Having clear goals and objectives was nominated almost twice as often as the next four factors, which were support from senior management, adequate funds or resources, a realistic schedule and end-user commitment (2002:7). The managers we interviewed nominated similar factors, but also placed emphasis on the need for long-term vision, sustainability of outcomes, and the problem of cultural fit between the project and the organisation. One respon-dent identified achieving change as both the key goal of projects in his organisation, and a key motivator: 'People have been able to abandon the sense of helplessness because they see projects are a way of getting some resources and bringing the tools to make changes that they want to make.'

The published studies typically give a dizzying list of requirements for success, often without any sense of the relationships between them. For example, they often nominate 'top management support' and 'adequate resources' among the most important (e.g. White and Fortune 2002). But these are not independent factors—if you have top management support, then you have a good chance of getting adequate resources; the reverse is also true.

Another limitation of the listing of success factors is that the diversity of projects, organisations and industries from which they are drawn means that it is virtually impossible to have a list that includes every success factor and, conversely, every list will have many factors that are not relevant to a given project. If an analysis of success factors is to be useful in practice, it must organise the wealth of possible elements into categories that make sense, and it must clarify the cause and effect relationships between factors.

Framework for success

Drawing on our research on current project management practice in the sector, and our own experience, we have tried to encapsulate the main insights and strategies needed by organisations and project managers to ensure that they use project management methods well and get value from their projects. We have developed a model, adapted from some important work by Belassi and Tukel (1996), which attempts to categorise the success factors meaningfully, and distinguish between underlying organisational and environmental factors and direct project variables.

We think this model helps to make sense of what is going on in the human services sector, and that it will be useful for project planners, decision makers and managers in several ways. It can be used as a framework for checking that key issues have been addressed in project planning and design, for understanding the implications of emerging problems and developing remedial action, for evaluation of project success and failure, and of how the organisation's overall project capacity might be improved. It could also be used by those who design funding programs and submission guidelines for projects—as a check to ensure that the requirements and criteria they include are consistent with funding successful projects.

The model (see Figure 1) has two major components. The 'project factors' on the right-hand side represent the direct determinants, or the reality of what happens with projects—what you can see happening on the ground, the project experience. These features, while critical to project success in their own right, are at least partly outcomes of the interplay of the 'underlying factors' on the left-hand side. The underlying factors are the conditions or enablers that together influence the project experience and outcomes, and are grouped in two categories or levels—factors in the sector, and characteristics of the organisation.

Figure 1: A model for project success factors

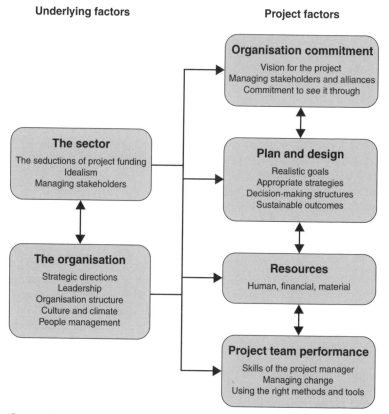

Source: Adapted from Belassi and Tukel (1996)

This framework proposes four main categories of direct determinants of project success:

- *Commitment:* Is the organisation serious, is there a vision for the project and commitment to see it through? Is there commitment to manage the impact on stakeholders and partners?
- *Plan and design:* Is the project plan feasible, with achievable goals, strategies that can work, good decision-making structures and outcomes that can be sustained?
- *Resources:* Are skilled people, enough money and the right material resources organised?
- *Project team:* Does the project team work well, is it able to manage the change required by the project and to communicate effectively with stakeholders?

We have divided the underlying factors into two major areas.

- *The sector:* This is the environmental context in which organisations, and thus their projects, sit. We have identified three major factors here: the first is the role of government, the second is idealism and the public good ethos; the third is the often contradictory forces of strategy versus opportunism.
- *The organisation:* The characteristics of the organisation include strategic directions, leadership, the organisational structure, and culture and people management practices.

The underlying factors which influence success or failure might be less amenable to change, at least for the purposes of a single project, and perhaps not at all. However, the logic of the framework is that attention to these issues—for example, thinking carefully about the 'fit' between the organisation's culture and the project, recognising the industrial issues that the project is likely to encounter and the likely stakeholder concerns—will enable organisations to choose projects, and pursue them, with a maximum chance of success. The industry and organisational factors which enable or constrain project success are discussed in Chapter 2.

SUMMARY

- Projects are a way of achieving one-off purposes, and there is a wealth of methods and tools available to support this work.

- The invention of the role of the project manager was a significant breakthrough, highlighting the importance of setting up the right roles and authority to ensure that projects have the needed resources.
- Most of the existing literature has been designed for engineering, IT and manufacturing industries; this book seeks to fill a gap for the human services industry.
- Projects are being used more and more frequently in a world of constant change and increasing complexity, but health and community service organisations are encountering some particular challenges in getting the anticipated value from their project work and in managing their project portfolios.
- These challenges include making strategic decisions about which projects to pursue, managing change, establishing clear and feasible project goals, providing effective leadership and skilled project teams, choosing the right tools and achieving sustainable outcomes.
- The available critiques of project management have relevance to the sector, and argue for modification of the mainstream methods to suit the needs of the sector (hence this book).
- The determinants of project success have been identified in an extensive literature. We present a framework for understanding success factors and how they relate to each other, focusing on the underlying factors in the sector and in organisations, and their impact on direct project management factors like adequate resources and top management support.

2

THE PROJECT CONTEXT:
THE SECTOR AND THE
ORGANISATION

In Chapter 1, we presented a brief analysis of the current challenges facing health and community service organisations in their project management practice. We also introduced a model for success. In this chapter, we develop the model further by exploring some of the characteristics of the sector that shape its project work and the organisational factors which enhance (or constrain) the capability for project success.

We suggest that despite the difficulties and challenges facing health and community service organisations, managers can create the conditions for project success, and focus on the practicalities of making it happen. To this end we propose key criteria for identifying and enabling potentially successful projects.

THE SECTOR CHALLENGE: PROJECTS AND STRATEGY

In recent years there has been a strong focus on improving management in the health and community services sector and on the particular features of the industry that impact on management practice. For our purposes these features can be narrowed down to four dimensions, all of which are relevant to project management success.

First, in most Western countries, the sector is largely government funded, and thereby subject to the vagaries of government policy change and direction setting. Even the private sector is significantly influenced by government policy. While this situation creates opportunities for growth it can also limit the strategic choice of organisations to set their own directions, and also requires senior managers to focus on balancing the demands of government with those of their own organisation.

Second, the industry is dynamic and parts of the sector are enmeshed in rapid technological and scientific development and change. These developments create opportunities for doing things better and can unleash the passion, energy and commitment needed to do so. However, they can also lead to key staff pulling in opposite and sometimes contradictory directions. Managers are often subjected to increasing demands for service development and resource allocation at a time of decreasing budgets and resources.

Third, this is a people-rich industry, with many tertiary-educated staff used to exercising a certain amount of professional independence, organised into powerful professional and trade union groups. This situation can lead to the 'contested ground' we discussed in Chapter 1, with some sections of the workforce agitating for change and others with something to lose digging in or refusing to engage.

Finally, the growth of the consumer movement has led to another powerful interest group which increasingly expects to have a voice in decision making at various levels. Added to this is the fact that health and community care are very politicised, attracting media attention and front-page headlines if things go wrong.

Against this background it is not surprising that our research indicates that managers in health and community service organisations experience some particular challenges in identifying and controlling their project agendas, in ensuring that the projects they do undertake are successful, and that their projects contribute to overall organisation strategy. By organisation strategy, we mean the chosen methods by which the organisation's purpose (often documented as 'vision and mission statements') is to be pursued and implemented. By making strategic choices between possible courses of action, the organisation determines what services or activities it will conduct, and how it will do so. One of the leadership challenges is then to mobilise the resources of the organisation towards success in the chosen areas of activity, and to avoid dissipating resources in activities which are not 'mission critical', as one manager we interviewed expressed it.

This challenge is not unique to the health and community services sector, but seems to have particular causes and effects in the sector exacerbated by the four features described above. Flowing from these features we have identified three major influences which have particular relevance to the sector's overall approach to projects: the seductions of project funding; idealism and the public good ethos; and managing the powerful stakeholders.

THE SEDUCTIONS OF PROJECT FUNDING

Governments and other funders have a major impact on the project portfolios of health and community service organisations. While this is true in both the private and public sectors, it is more acute for government-funded agencies. The impact of government has risen over recent years in many ways, partly through the increased use of project funding as a strategy for encouraging change in practice and models of care, and for enhancing government's ability to monitor and control agencies.

Why there is so much project funding

A little history is relevant here. In the latter part of the twentieth century, governments in many countries attempted to draw a clear separation between the business of deciding what human services to provide (characterised as the purchasing of services) and the business of providing those services. The so-called purchaser/provider split was part of the reform of public administration known as managerialism or New Public Management (Pollitt 1995). It was based on a desire to gain greater control of the supply side of health and community services and on the principle that governments, rather than doctors, hospitals, or health and community service agencies, should decide more precisely what services would be paid for by the taxpayer.

With this movement came increasing activism on the part of central health and human service authorities in relation to the standards and quality of services, and in the drive for innovation in methods of service delivery. One result has been the proliferation of project-based funding programs, which essentially fund and reward innovation in compliance with government policy directions. Some of these programs, like the National Demonstration Hospitals Program (NDHP) in Australia, and other state-based programs, have been very successful in driving change. For example, increased use of day surgery and day-of-surgery admission to hospitals has been driven by financial pressure, but enabled partly by the availability of project funding (through NDHP and a range of state-based programs).

Government as project funder: risks and rewards

For the most part these funding programs are valuable, and have enabled cash-strapped agencies to acquire and use resources for change and innovation. By this method the funder, rather than the agency itself, makes the tough decision that a pot of money will not be spent on direct service delivery, or at least not on 'business as usual' services.

Agencies in their turn develop skills in presenting their priorities in the clothing of the funder's policy goals, while still retaining focus on their own goals as well. However, the increasing use of project funding as an incentive for change and innovation brings a real risk that funding itself will become a major driver of the agency's attention, energy and resources, usurping the role that strategic directions and business strategies should play. Two-thirds of the people we interviewed identified this as a serious problem. For example, a manager in a large health agency noted: 'I think we actually just responded to the government and then in hindsight tried to make the best of it . . . the government is a bit too prescriptive.'

Similarly in primary care, a representative of a general practice organisation noted the danger of losing focus through a major funded project the organisation was involved in. It 'tended to dominate and detract from other programs and so it really was an exercise and a lesson in the importance of coming back to your original strategic plan, your customers, and not getting carried off on a tangent just because there might be some additional funding'.

On the other hand, one large hospital reported that the availability of funding programs, and the hospital's increasing success in gaining project funding, had enabled the hospital to drive its own agenda, a capacity which had grown in five years from a standing start (virtually no projects) to a sophisticated and successful project strategy. 'We have tried to support clinical people finding solutions to clinical problems rather than finding the answers for them.'

Resourcing projects is an important contribution by government which enhances the ability of organisations to innovate (Dwyer and Leggat 2002) and improve their effectiveness. One senior manager in a government department explained the three reasons that his department funded hospitals to innovate. First, innovation funding, which costs a tiny proportion of the total funding for service delivery, was seen as an investment in good practice and innovation. Second, the department was seen as having an interest in and a responsibility to assist the biggest and most vexed part of the human services system. Finally, the innovation funding was seen as giving the department a 'foot in the door', and better contact with the realities of service delivery, 'almost as a training ground for some of our people'.

Mismatches between the project agenda of government and the business strategy of agencies can be a source of significant risk. The development of infrastructure is a case in point—the introduction of new IT systems, and capital building projects, are often run jointly by the government funder and the recipient agency, for good reasons. However, problems of different agendas, timing and scale emerge. As one CEO who had lost control of decision making about key administrative IT systems put it: 'Nobody in their right mind would change all of their computing systems in one year . . . and yet we're doing it.'

A general practice (GP) division described their projects as detracting from core business: 'The feedback we were getting was that the GPs weren't seeing much [assistance with everyday problems]. They felt that the Division wasn't making any difference in their lives and therefore their patient or their community.' This organisation decided not to do major projects 'without first of all ensuring that what was happening back at home base or at the core of your existence was being addressed properly'.

One hospital manager noted: 'All projects walk a fine line between interfering with the day-to-day business and the focus of people on their day-to-day business and giving them an out to go and do some other things that might be a bit more glamorous. I actually think it is a very big issue for nursing, and I think a lot of nurses who are dissatisfied with nursing *per se* see this as an alternative avenue.'

General practice divisions also commented on the 'project feed method' which was the predominant funding method used by the Australian federal government in the 1990s, describing it as 'Darwinistic—you can pick the things you really like and aggressively pursue them'. However, this commentator also believed that the government's new method of funding divisions, on the basis of agreed strategic and business plans, gave it more room to 'rule the strategy'. That is, rather than the haphazard influence on strategy which arises from the grab-bag approach, the funder gained greater scope to control strategy by requiring the submission of strategic plans before allocating funds. Whether that scope is used or not is a separate question. It could also be argued that this method simply promotes good governance by ensuring that some sort of strategic direction exists.

Although we have outlined the problems generated by government influence on project decision making, it must be noted that project funding has also served as a vital source of innovation resources, and that service delivery agencies have often made wise use of the available funding. As the senior public servant quoted above observed: 'On balance the hospitals have been well served . . . they tend to use those resources very well. My observation is that the hospital sector had very little access to discretionary resources . . . By and large they work out what they want to use that small precious amount of money for and they use it well.'

IDEALISM AND THE PUBLIC GOOD ETHOS

Idealism is an issue for the management of individual projects in health and community services, as well as for the management of project portfolios—and not only in the public sector. Commitment to the public good ethos is seen in heroic effort against the odds, in acceptance of ambiguity and complexity, and also in the difficulty experienced by many health and community service organisations in choosing priorities among competing needs or options. The process of decision making about new initiatives in agencies, in which judgments about which worthy project to sacrifice and which to approve, is often prolonged, emotional, politicised and less strategic than managers would like to admit.

Perhaps the business culture that produced modern project management is more pragmatic, with more concrete goals and more direct methods of pursuing them, than is the health and community services culture. It is hard to imagine the slogan 'faster, better, cheaper', with its implication of uncomplicated acceptance of a clear and concrete goal, becoming a rallying cry in human services. Ideals like 'equity, access, quality' are both more familiar, and more abstract and complex.

Idealism and commitment can also be a source of resistance to change. The 'missionary organisation' (Mintzberg 1991) is one which pursues values-based goals (like relieving suffering or reducing inequality) and attracts staff who are personally driven by those goals. Their commitment, however, may lead them to resist what they perceive as incorrect interpretations of the mission. When this tendency is linked to self-interest (for example, a proposed change to a model of service which will require change in patterns of work) it can be a powerful force. Any attempt to change the way that things are done can be seen as an attack on the fundamental values and philosophies of the organisation which will undermine service quality and commitment to consumers. We return to this point in Chapter 6 when we explore the management of change.

We have found in our teaching, as well as in the interviews for this book, that health and community services staff can have difficulty accepting some of the basic features of the project method: the limited goals, the emphasis on concrete 'deliverables', and the importance of questions like 'will it be finished by the end of next month?'.

A senior manager in a large health organisation explained why his organisation experiences difficulty containing their project portfolio: 'Overestimating what can be done is the first thing. Lack of focus, probably discipline and structure, to actually make sure that there is scrutiny on things before they go ahead; and a little bit of a sense that it has got to be shared around, a bit of competitiveness as well.' He advocated recognition of the need 'to be a bit more rigorous and accept that we actually should do a couple of things better [rather] than doing a lot of things and maybe not really doing that much at all'.

While there are many situations in which achievement of goals would be enhanced by the use of project management, there are also problems of misapplication of the method. The experience we have characterised as managing an elephant (see Case 1) illustrates the problem of trying to apply project management to tasks which cannot be adequately supported by this method.

Case 1: Is this work a project or an elephant?

One of the more positive developments in human services in recent years has occurred in the area of early childhood services—the growing recognition of the life-long importance for children of getting a good start, and the development of new and effective ways of supporting families and children to ensure that they do.

A project manager in a large government agency described the challenges of her major project based on this new direction. She was tasked to develop a coordinated, cross-portfolio approach which would require shifting both the priorities and the methods of funders and providers of early childhood services to the new approach. She was struggling with inter-departmental committees, the coordination of funding lines and the need for change in some long established and highly valued community services.

Not surprisingly, she found the language and methods of project management inadequate and incorrectly focused for her task. She knew and accepted that she would never have the authority to 'project manage' what she described as a process of social policy change. She would have to rely on alliance building, clever tactics, good will and the power of small successes to 'seduce' the sceptics. And she knew that such shifts would be gradually achieved, and that success would not necessarily be promoted by sharing the grand vision too early. Her resilience in the face of slipping timelines, road-blocks, differing expectations by key stakeholders and the occasional disappointments of ineffective executive support was inspiring. Her commitment to the larger goal, as well as the support of some leaders inside and outside the bureaucracy, sustained her.

On reflection, she decided that she had the management of several projects and one large elephant*. Project management was useful for the tasks of demonstrating and evaluating models of service delivery inspired and funded through this work, but the overarching work itself required different concepts and approaches.

*This term was used in the 1990s in the quality movement to describe quality improvement projects that were too big to be manageable.

MANAGING THE KEY STAKEHOLDERS

One of the most difficult challenges in project management in the sector is managing the key stakeholders and influential people and groups who often have different and competing agendas. Often the person with the loudest voice or strongest personality or most important position can take a project in an entirely different direction on a whim or a 'good idea'. At the industry level there are a number of key stakeholders who might become involved in a project, perhaps through being part of a steering or advisory committee, being a project funder or part of the project process. Different professional and trade union groups may have their own sectoral interests that are beyond the scope of the project but that can stymie change and derail projects, sometimes deliberately, but sometimes because their adherence to their own agenda does not allow them to see any alternatives.

Governments through their role as funders are also key stakeholders and government agencies can change their minds and alter their policy directions well into the project lifecycle, due to a change in government, a change of minister or key personnel, or because more important priorities come along. Governments are also susceptible to public opinion and political lobbying, and a project that has potential for unpopularity is vulnerable if a strong opposition mobilises against it.

Consumers are another important stakeholder group which can be difficult to engage, involve and manage. Consumers with a chronic condition might be too ill to involve for very long in a project, other consumers might be transitory and move on to other interests. Consumers can often become disillusioned by their experiences in committees or reference groups. Perhaps their expectations are so high that they are never likely to be realised, or more likely, they feel disempowered by the attitudes of the professionals involved in the project management process.

On the other hand, a lot has been learned in recent years about both goals and effective approaches to involving consumers, and our informants identified some real contributions to project success. Consumers often bring practical ideas for service improvement; they can become powerful ambassadors for the agency, and help to enhance relationships between users and providers of care.

In many situations the influence of powerful people pulling in different directions leads to a stakeholder paralysis where nothing gets done and people become angry and frustrated. Case 2 gives an alternative method for engaging stakeholders in the decision-making process. Careful attention should be given to the management of stakeholders on a number of levels, and this issue is addressed in Chapter 5.

Case 2: Getting beyond stakeholder paralysis

The leadership group of a major teaching hospital faced the challenge of reorganising their operating theatre structure to enable the formation of effective teams and thereby improve the service delivered by the theatres to their users, the surgeons and patients. A member of the leadership group, who had rich experience of change projects such as this becoming bogged down through the creation of steering committees on which all stakeholder interests were represented, proposed a radical alternative. He suggested that the CEO and a senior clinician (who was identified as not having a structural stake in the question) act as a panel of review and design the best possible structure. The outcome of their deliberations should be brought back to the group for endorsement and then implemented.

To the CEO's surprise, this suggestion was universally supported, and the two-person team (with project officer support) proceeded to invite submissions and conduct interviews, to commission a small literature review and prepare a short report. They recommended major structural change to achieve a situation in which all major groups working in the theatres (excluding the surgeons who were defined as 'users' of theatre services) would report to a theatre suite manager and work in multi-disciplinary teams.

The CEOs experience was that the process of submissions and interviews enabled the various staff groups to tell some of the real stories and identify the obstacles to improved service; and enabled both providers and users to identify the outcomes they sought rather than focusing on the 'ownership' issues. The report was readily accepted, and the momentum for constructive change carried through to successful implementation. Key success

---

factors were identified as a level of objectivity to focus on the goals, and the trust of those affected, trust which had been enhanced by the process which was transparent while providing safety for those who participated. In the end, stakeholder interests were heard and incorporated, but the paralysis often encountered in the stakeholder committee structure was avoided.

PROJECT CAPABILITY: THE ORGANISATIONAL CHALLENGE

Factors that influence project success at the level of the organisation are largely about capability: the characteristics that enable organisations to mount successful projects or which constrain their project success. The health and community services field is made up of diverse organisations, each with its own unique project management features and experiences. However, there are a number of common success factors that operate at the level of the organisation as a whole: strategic directions, leadership, structure, culture and approaches to the management of people. Focus on these factors is an important strategy; managers need to recognise these underlying issues, and anticipate and manage their potential positive or negative impact.

Setting strategic directions and sticking to them

The impact of the strategic direction of the organisation on its project success depends on two elements: alignment of projects to the plan, and strength of the plan. First, the success of a project will depend partly on how it aligns with the organisation's strategies for achieving its basic purpose or mission. Second, as well as alignment, the relative strength of the strategic direction (how strongly and broadly it is supported throughout the organisation) will impact on the ability of the organisation to muster coordinated support for a key project. The reverse is also true: if the strategic plan is a weak instrument, it is less of a barrier for an irrelevant project that is not aligned or relevant to the plan.

'Coming back to the plan', as one CEO described it, was an important theme for the managers we interviewed. But it is difficult to use the organisation's strategic plan as a test for the priority of particular funding opportunities if the plan is not strongly understood and valued by the majority of influential people or groups in the organisation. We found this to be a major source of difficulties with managing the project portfolio, and not only in human services. A large study in the US pharmaceutical industry, for example, found that managers in many of the firms surveyed singled out the organisation's inability to prioritise effectively as a key weakness, caused by 'countervailing organisational special interests' that are able to resist the portfolio level decisions of senior management (Case 1998:593).

Most health and community service organisations have a strategic directions document of some kind, but for many the thinking behind it and commitment to its intended outcomes are not shared strongly enough throughout the organisation to allow it to drive decision making from board level down. To look at this another way, the problem is not that there are no strategic directions, but rather that there are several competing and perhaps contradictory ones.

Internal politics is an ongoing reality—the interests of individuals, units and teams within the organisation will not always align with the organisation's broader interests or strategies, and the result is both a leadership and management problem. Neither managers nor projects can change this reality, part of what is sometimes called the 'shadow side' of organisations (Egan 1994), but there are strategies for managing it. Strategic plans can be designed to recognise and better align the interests of important internal stakeholders with those of the organisation as a whole. They can also be used in such a way as to channel 'political' activity out of the corridors and into structured priority-setting processes. We return to this difficult question in Chapter 6.

The theory of professional bureaucracy

In human services, the problem of strategic direction has some particular characteristics, and the theory of 'professional bureaucracy' as a form of organisation (Mintzberg and Quinn 1991) is helpful for understanding it. This form is typified by hospitals, universities, large accounting and law firms—that is, large organisations which employ highly skilled and high-status professionals to provide services tailored to the needs of individual patients or clients. This form of organisation, which relies on disseminated decision making rather than strong control from the top, also relies on having a relatively stable and friendly environment.

Organisations of this type have been under great pressure to change since the 1980s, in particular to enable increased managerial control and thereby the ability to act in a more coordinated way, and to make and implement decisions quickly. But the co-existence of several competing strategic agendas persists as an enduring feature of the culture of human service organisations (including government departments), and makes it hard for them to establish overarching strategic directions which are accepted broadly enough in practice.

This characteristic may also have some advantages—for example, enabling clinicians to pursue clinical innovations not foreseen in the strategic plan, or limiting the practical impact of adverse policy decisions. One of the tried and true techniques of resistance in bureaucracies is to go slow on implementing a decision which is seen as wrong, in order to limit the damage while waiting for the decision to be reversed. However, two of the disadvantages of competing agendas are that they make it harder for the organisation to achieve a unified direction and for the leadership level to impose discipline on the project agenda.

Ad hoc decision making

Our informants expressed this problem in many different ways, but all of them referred to it. One government department manager said that the determinant of whether projects were supported was, to a degree, 'about how loud the voice is and where the voice is coming from'. A community service manager was more blunt: 'I'd like to be able to say that we have a very defined strategic plan and we work to that but we don't.'

The CEO of a major hospital acknowledged that the organisation was just beginning to use its strategic directions document—'What we are trying to do is get some business rigour into our decisions with regard to where the organisation is and where it is going'—and she estimated a success rate (that is, of selecting, shaping or excluding a project on this basis) of about 60 per cent. Another large organisation reported a real problem with the inability to discipline decision making about projects, including at the executive level, because of the existence of a large number of internal stakeholders with radically different agendas.

A primary care manager highlighted the problem of ad hoc decision making at the governance level: 'The decisions were really driven by personal decision making amongst board members and their view of was it a good idea or a bad idea.'

In this section, we have discussed the problems for the sector of constraints on strategic choice, and a culture that doesn't support a strong unified focus on strategic direction. But it is also true that some organisations do achieve the ability to pursue their chosen strategies, with a significant positive impact on project capability.

LEADERSHIP AT EVERY LEVEL

One of the major requirements for project success identified by our respondents was effective leadership. Leadership to ensure staff 'own' the project and understand how it fits into the overall direction of the organisation is critical. As most interviewees commented, if you haven't got high level endorsement and championing, it is very hard to make even a great idea work. 'They need a fairly savvy person actually driving the project— the hands-on person—but you also need high-level endorsement and if you haven't got that then, I think, it is very difficult to make a project work.'

People we interviewed also commented on the difficult leadership task of both generating commitment and simultaneously imposing discipline on project activity, a task which is challenging for all of the reasons outlined earlier in this chapter. This task applies at all levels of the organisation, from the board of directors to project team members.

CAPABLE STRUCTURES

We have argued earlier that many projects in human service organisations are about improvement and innovation. More specifically, they are often directed to changing the systems and processes by which the organisation produces its services (both services to end users—the clients, communities and patients; and the internal support services that enable the former to work). This means that the majority of projects engage with the business of more than one department or team within the organisation, and will almost inevitably cut across normal ongoing departmental operations in some way.

This raises two important issues about organisation structure. First, how do projects, and project teams, relate to the ongoing operational structures of the organisation? And second, are some structures more suitable for organisations that actively use projects to enhance their effectiveness?

The structure and the team

Alsene (1998), in a review of the project management literature, outlines three types of structures for the management of projects: functional, project and matrix. In the *functional structure*, the project team is made up primarily of people who work within an operational division, who take on the project work in addition to other responsibilities and retain their normal reporting lines. Overall responsibility for the project is generally allocated to the functional unit that contributes the most to the project. A *project structure* is one where the team members are released from their regular duties (full- or part-time) and report to a project manager who in turn reports to a senior manager (or steering committee). The project manager is autonomous from the functional structure of the organisation. A *matrix structure* is one in which team members remain under the authority of their normal functional supervisor while being coordinated by a project manager with a different reporting line.

Alsene reports a general view that there is no 'one best way' and that the choice depends on the project, with the functional structure being the most common. Resistance to change and the tendency of line managers not to relinquish power readily are pervasive reasons for the apparent preference to work through existing structures. However, using three case studies from industry, Alsene goes on to argue that the project structure is the best for projects which aim to bring about internal change of any significant scope. This structure frees up the individuals to focus on the priorities of the project; it minimises problems of conflicting loyalties and maximises the opportunity for multi-disciplinary problem solving and organisational learning.

Experience in the organisations we surveyed tends to support this conclusion. The common experience of failure (or disappointing results) in change and innovation projects can often be seen to proceed from the failure to free the project itself from the entrenched interests which can be predicted to resist change. One informant expressed this as 'the power of organisational culture and the maintenance of bureaucratic processes over the efficiency of a project'.

The creation of effective project team structures may only be achievable when this method is broadly understood by the stakeholders who must relinquish control, and when they can be satisfied that their legitimate interests will be protected (the PRINCE model in particular includes a nice way of approaching this task—see Chapter 5). Success may also be supported through location of control of the project team with a person or unit seen to be neutral to the competing interests affected by the project and skilled in managing the potential conflicts. This tends to argue for careful consideration of the potential wins and losses in advance, and placement of major change projects centrally, away from competing operational areas.

Managing by projects

For some organisations, the projects *are* the main services or products; that is, the delivery of a series of projects is the organisation's purpose and all of the organisation's major functions are conceived and managed as projects.

In industries such as aircraft manufacturing, where tailored products are made to fill specific orders, 'project network structures' are advocated (Ayas 1996). The line management structure is based on programs; that is, groupings of projects or potential projects by type, required expertise, production process or location. Major projects may be managed through a constellation of small teams, with membership and management changing in response to the needs of the project. While this type of organisation is largely not applicable to human service agencies, it is relevant for organisations with major roles in social advocacy, health promotion or representation of interest groups, and we found some evidence of the project structure in at least part of some agencies we studied.

To a certain extent, primary care organisations such as community health and women's health services have operated in this way for many years, but through necessity rather than choice. These agencies were often structured around a small amount of core funding and over time became an umbrella for a disparate collection of projects and programs. While the project-based structures they developed had certain advantages in terms of flexibility and the speed with which agencies could respond to new initiatives and demands, they also had their limitations. Often there was conflict between the different project teams and groupings, and loss of commitment to the goals, vision and philosophy of the parent organisation. There was also often a sense of crisis or insecurity within the agency as it struggled for funding opportunities to keep its staff and community profile.

The Australian divisions of general practice in the late 1990s had the experience of managing by projects, when this was the funding method, and their organisations showed some features of the project structure. A division manager who was perhaps influenced by this experience also advocated a project approach to renewal, that is, that the organisation should include in its project portfolio a regular program of re-examining the departments that 'just float along for years ... A good organisation chooses as part of its strategic process its most vulnerable piece, its oldest piece, and says this year we are going to revisit that and reshape it'.

When most activities in the organisation, or a major part of it, are structured as short-term interventions uniquely tailored to particular client or community groups, fluid accountability lines based on the project network structure may be both effective and achievable.

The problem of a member of staff having two bosses is raised in the literature, but is not unique to project structures. As Healy (1997:30) points out, the two-boss situation is a result of the dual need for project staff to focus on the project and maintain their specialist skills: 'The two-boss dilemma is here to stay.'

Managing groups of projects

For many organisations in our study, projects were an ongoing feature of their work, and they had developed some ongoing capacity to coordinate and support them. One government department and two of the larger agencies had established small units to coordinate and support their project work (in some cases along with other functions like planning and development). The project unit roles typically included conducting major projects, training staff in project management, developing templates and tools for staff to use, coordinating responses to funding opportunities, recruiting project staff and acting as advisers to project teams.

Several other agencies had internal units dedicated to quality or clinical improvement, which typically took on some of the roles listed above, but with a focus on clinical practice change. A large teaching hospital used a project coordinating committee, made up of members of the executive and other senior corporate staff, which monitored and supported projects throughout the organisation. Smaller organisations tended to have the management team or the entire staff involved in the decision making, coordination and support of projects.

The staff working in project units had varied backgrounds, including experience as consultants. One leading project manager had cut her teeth on a major organisation change project where she was the in-house member seconded to a team of consultants—she went on to work in one of the large consultancy firms and then returned to a health service as a project manager. The typical path for in-house project staff seems to be an initial opportunity to learn as part of a team, the discovery of ability and interest in project work, followed by further development and the building of impressive track records.

BUILDING A PROJECT MANAGEMENT CULTURE

It has become fashionable to characterise organisational cultures according to their relevance for particular goals. Thus management writers and consultants advocate for 'quality culture', 'innovation culture', 'learning culture' or 'high performance culture', and project management writers are part of this trend (e.g. O'Kelly and Maxwell 2001).

Organisation culture is a much-discussed but ill-defined concept which makes intuitive sense to most people who have worked in organisations but is hard to study and perhaps even harder to manipulate. By culture, we mean the unwritten values and rules that are understood and endorsed by the staff (or important subgroups) and therefore govern 'how things are done around here'.

According to our research, organisations with a culture which is supportive of project success have three key characteristics: they have an ability to handle change; they have the ability to incorporate new knowledge, that is, to learn; and there is a disseminated awareness among staff of the project method and how it can be used. These characteristics, particularly the first two, are generally also seen as part of those other desired cultures (high performance, quality, etc.), and there is a vast literature on these questions (see, for example, Leggat and Dwyer 2003 for a review of the literature on innovation and culture). The implication of the concept of project management culture is that an organisation seeking to improve its project success will benefit from enhancing those aspects of its culture which support change, project capability and the ability to learn.

O'Kelly and Maxwell (2001) argue enthusiastically for the adoption of a project management culture in health care, particularly in relation to the implementation of clinical governance in the UK. For these authors, a project management culture implies an ability to initiate change and get things done in a manageable way through the use of project teams. These teams are comprised of people who reach across the traditional professional boundaries in health care to focus on patients and improvements in service delivery.

Organisational structures as well as cultures can enhance or undermine a project management culture. For example, organisations that encourage and nurture multi-disciplinary teams and genuine partnerships between professional groups are likely to have a more open approach to doing things differently. A project management culture can also mean that ideas are encouraged, good ideas supported and actions are followed up, with clear reporting and accountability structures.

Halligan and Donaldson (2001) also take a project management approach to the task of introducing clinical governance in the UK, and outline their definition of a project management culture. They argue the need for effective leadership that empowers teamwork and creates an open, questioning climate. They suggest that high quality and performance in health care depend on ordinary people doing extraordinary things. To enable this to happen they argue for education and training, practices which value staff, management being seen to tackle the problems that staff identify, good technical support and a culture free of blame.

The culture of government departments has an influence on their ability to carry out good projects and their funding and supervision of others. The people we interviewed felt that government departments can be more atomised than other organisations, and the staff distanced from practical outcomes of their work. They sometimes incorporate many different interest groups in conflict with each other. The power of personalities is seen as an important component of organisational culture, as is the power of the culture to maintain bureaucratic processes at the expense of the [efficiency of a] project. We also found evidence that the challenge of developing a project management culture within central human service authorities is recognised and work is underway to identify barriers and enablers.

The organisations we studied identified several cultural characteristics that can get in the way of project success. One project director noted: 'We are a very action-orientated culture and people don't spend the time in planning and thinking through a vision before they just get in and do. It's absolutely notable how many times an issue will be raised and the next minute you know, three people have gone away and are doing things. Nobody has actually checked whether they are doing the right things.'

The prescriptions for enhancing culture quoted above may seem like forlorn hopes to embattled project managers and senior managers in organisations. Culture change may be difficult and slow, but attention to culture is useful for two reasons. First, even difficult and slow processes have to begin somewhere, and projects can make a significant contribution to culture change. Second, the savvy project manager needs to see clearly, and work with and around, the cultural barriers they can't change.

PEOPLE MANAGEMENT AND ORGANISATION DEVELOPMENT

Attention to the people side of organisations, in developing and sustaining their project capacity, is also vital—finding and keeping good project managers, and embedding the skills of project management as part of their organisational knowledge.

Almost all the project management literature and all our interviewees spoke about the importance of having the right staff. This will not be achieved by making people into project managers either because they have a good idea and want to be the one to implement it, or because you have nothing else for them to do and need to find them a job. A project director quoted earlier in this chapter also expressed concern about the use of projects as an escape from the rigours of mainstream work. Some organisations take what may be the easy way out and 'buy in' project managers from outside, either as consultants or as temporary employees. This can work well but is not always a satisfactory solution—consultants can be expensive, they might not fit in with organisational culture easily and they might not be very good despite their glowing references and marketing publicity. The same with temporary project managers—by the time you find out that they haven't really got the skills you thought they had, you are halfway through the project.

It may be more strategic to identify and keep good project managers within the organisation. Several organisations we studied had introduced training and development programs in project management. These programs can be seen as an important part of organisation development and capacity building. One manager explained that capacity building was an important part of her organisation's direction: 'We have focused a lot of professional development around broad in-service training so that we are backing our projects up, particularly the health promotion ones, with staff education, capacity building and support.' Skills that are seen as valuable for project management such as communication, negotiation, facilitation and conflict management are valuable for all managers. These skills, along with others such as managing teams and managing change, can be an important part of a wider management development program.

The temporary nature of projects, and particularly the timing of project funding, also means that organisations need to focus on embedding the learning and skills gained through the project, and retaining corporate knowledge. This can be difficult if project managers are contract staff and their contracts come to an end, when 'the intellectual history and corporate memory depart', unless an emphasis is placed on adequate handover [and] documentation. Many organisations give little thought to these issues until it is too late.

PROJECTS IN GOVERNMENT DEPARTMENTS

Government looms large in project management in the public sector, with central health and human service authorities being involved at several levels. Their programs generate and direct a lot of the project activity in service delivery agencies. They also conduct or commission a large number of projects as part of their own responsibilities, and they too experience difficulties managing their project portfolios. Government, like human service agencies, is an area where the ideal of fixed goals and timelines is particularly hard to achieve, because of constant 'responding to processes and pressure and a changing environment', as one senior public servant put it.

Much of the work of staff in central health authorities (departments of health, aged care, community or human services) can be defined as projects. The development of policies and standards, and the operation of a submission and approval process to allocate short-term funds, are common examples. One senior public servant described his role as a combination of program management and policy development, and characterised both aspects as being largely project based. The processes of project definition and project approval have a political as well as a bureaucratic component, and the birth of projects may be particularly complicated in sensitive and newly emerging policy areas. Projects emerge from the interplay of political decision making, interpretations at the governance level of the department and less elevated operational processes.

A consultant we interviewed put it strongly—'government manages by projects'—and identified three main reasons for the extensive use of external consultants. First, at state level, reductions in the size of the public sector workforce, and the resultant loss of 'good people', have made it harder for departments to contribute to policy development. Executives must often choose between 'treading water' (and thereby making little progress on major issues) or using outsourced intellectual capability. Second, external consultants are used for 'leapfrogging quick change', especially in politically sensitive areas where major policy jigsaws need to be managed. Third, external players are seen as being more objective, while also bringing the benefit of the transfer of skills to departmental staff.

The Australian federal government is seen to tender projects for three major reasons: when it lacks the technical skills or critical mass for the work; to 'buy time' on issues people cannot or do not want to deal with; and to manage the difficult politics of national projects, where federal and state/territory governments must work together. The extensive use of external consultants is also seen to arise from the prevalence at the national level of 'career bureaucrats' who lack content expertise in any particular policy area.

The public servants we interviewed agreed that one of the difficulties for project managers in government is the absence (sometimes for good reason) of a clearly defined and agreed project goal. A senior public servant described major projects as 'emerging' when 'a process of sensitivity to policy-relevant issues gets to the point where you say we actually have to do some work'. It is in the nature of government that major projects will have 'some articulated goals and probably some other not-officially-articulated agendas as well'. This is an important problem for the practical project manager, but also for those who seek to allocate priority among competing projects.

In our research, some government departments were identified as being very sophisticated users of projects and as running project portfolios that strongly reflect key policy and strategic agenda. But it was also noted that organisations need a strong vision about 'where they're really going with major, policy-relevant projects in government', and that this is often lacking. This is particularly problematic when projects are mounted in sensitive areas of social policy, such as the interface between hospitals and aged care, or the development of a united approach to early intervention for the wellbeing of children.

One interviewee agreed that the government approach to project management 'is still fairly much around the project administration rather than the broader policy issues or the broader rationale including the social policy agenda'. It was also noted that examination of the processes of project development and priority-setting was not encouraged: 'How much you look internal to the organisation and how the organisation operates or influences outcomes is still I think pretty taboo.' Government departments also face particular barriers against engaging stakeholders. As one senior manager put it: 'If you moot changes, you unleash opposition from the forces of "no change"—then you certainly get instant feedback, but sometimes because all hell breaks loose.'

ORGANISATIONAL PROJECT STRATEGY

We have suggested that there are three major factors operating in the health and community services industry as a whole which underlie or impede project success—the influence of funding opportunities, the presence of key power groups, and the impact of idealism and commitment to broad social goals.

We have also suggested that there are five major organisational factors which determine the project capability of human

45

service organisations—strategic direction, leadership, structure and culture, and people management practices. In Part 2 of this book we turn to the models and methods of project management which are the immediate influences on project success, and which we have argued are supported or constrained by the industry and organisational factors outlined above. But first, we want to apply the industry and organisational analysis to the question of project strategy: the decisions organisations make about what project opportunities to pursue, and how they manage their overall project effort. In the rest of this chapter, we present some criteria for use in choosing projects in human service organisations—the organisation's 'project portfolio' is the sum of these choices.

THE PROJECT OR THE PLAN

'Well, if it's not in the plan, it doesn't get funded.' (*Hospital CEO*)

The rational planning approach to developing a project portfolio is embodied in the Project Management Body of Knowledge (Project Management Institute 2000) and reflected in many text-books (e.g. Haynes 1994; Dobson 1996; Rosenau 1998; Verzuh 1999). The strategic plan is the first step, followed by the development of programs of activity to implement the plan, and then the commissioning of projects to develop, enable, support or modify the activities. A further level of subprojects is used if size, complexity or staging require it. Thus programs are related to organisation strategy, and ongoing program management (for example, managing a fundraising program) is supported by project management (for example, staging a breast cancer ball).

The rational approach was reflected in the way some of our informants described their practice. Several had instituted organised methods for developing project proposals, designing criteria for their approval, ranking proposals against each other, selecting those to be approved (either for internal funding or to be included in bids for external funding) and resourcing and coordinating the resultant activities.

In larger organisations, this was generally at the program level—that is, a set of projects which were seen to be truly competing with each other for endorsement and resources within a division or program—rather than a comprehensive approach at the level of the organisation as a whole. Some smaller organisations used the latter approach to their advantage, ensuring coherence and manageability through a comprehensive annual priority-setting process.

Most of the managers we interviewed had experienced growing acceptance of the discipline of sticking to the strategic plan, often as a result of the pain of failing to do so. 'Our decision to do work which furthered our strategic direction was very deliberate because the organisation was being torn apart by a multi-directional project management way of working. We've been very disciplined about it. Constantly questioning and making people explain how their ideas further the strategic direction of the organisation.'

A community-based health service manager explained: 'We have developed business plans and everyone thinks they are a pain in the neck but they are beginning to see that we've now got a direction.' Another primary care manager put it like this: 'You have got to be more ruthless at that governance and conceptual and strategic level about does it actually take you forwards or not . . . we have got to say projects can't be developed, they can't get credibility in our organisation, if they are not mission critical.'

The rational planning method has many attractions, but often cannot be achieved. Our informants nominated several reasons why the strategic plan might not help at the time the decisions about individual projects have to be made. They include the strategic plan being up for review; that there is a new CEO and leadership team; that the strategic plan only deals with service delivery issues and is insufficient as a guide to prioritising project decisions in support areas.

In spite of these limitations, our research and the literature indicate that it is useful to cling to the plan as much as possible and to develop open, predictable, rational methods for prioritising projects. Taking this basic proposition as a starting point, the next question is to develop criteria and methods for managing the project portfolio. Case 3 recounts a profound experience of learning about the importance of the plan.

Case 3: A general practice division's project experience

The Brisbane North Division of General Practice did their project learning on a large scale. The former CEO describes a transformation in an organisation, which had itself existed only for a few years, when it took on a high-profile high-risk multi-million dollar project (the Coordinated Care Trial, 1998–2000). This experience was an important factor in shaping their identity and their organisation strategy.

Before the trial experience, decisions about which projects to select were driven by personal decision making among board members based on their personal views about the worth of the idea. After evaluating the impact of the trial ('successful but consuming'), Brisbane North developed a statement of strategic intent. They aimed to be 'at the cutting edge of health services reform for general practice/primary care', and resolved not to take on small projects, projects that couldn't be adequately resourced and, most importantly, projects that were not 'mission critical'.

The leadership group were fully committed to the strategic intent, and learned to make decisions about projects that would support their direction and develop their desired position as a leader in general practice innovation.

CRITERIA FOR CHOOSING THE PROJECT PORTFOLIO

The goal of selection of projects has been described as the search for 'a paddock of thoroughbreds' (Case 1998)—that is, each project should be well designed and capable of delivering the desired results. The criteria actually used for adopting projects into a portfolio will be unique to each organisation, and probably to the program or business area, and will change over time. Different criteria will get different weightings, sometimes overtly, sometimes covertly. Alignment with the organisation's strategic intent is often espoused as the major criterion, but decisions can always be influenced by other agendas, or simply a rush of enthusiasm. Having explicit criteria, and a rigorous process for applying them, is a safeguard against the influence of organisational politics or an excess of zeal, but not a guarantee. On the other hand, not having explicit criteria is an almost guaranteed method of ensuring that many of the wrong horses get into the paddock. The ideas presented below are based on the project success model developed in Chapter 1, and are expressed as generic templates or principles that might be used in designing criteria.

1. Will this project help to achieve our strategic goals, directly or indirectly?

We have said that this is really the starting point, but for many health and community service organisations the goals are so broad that even moderately skilled enthusiasts can make a case for almost anything under this sort of criterion. Goal-setting theory tells us that specific goals are more motivating than vague general ones (Latham and Locke 1979), and in this case specific strategic goals are more useful as criteria. If the strategic directions document or business plan is not specific enough, it can be modified into a state-ment of strategic goals for projects in the organisation, borrowing legitimacy from the strategic directions document while making it more readily useful for project portfolio management.

One hospital CEO we interviewed described her organisa-tion as essentially three separate businesses: clinical services, facility services and corporate services. She noted that their strategic directions statement was focused on clinical areas, and that for project decisions in the other areas she needed other goals. She opted to use a combination of the logical consequences of the clinical plan (for example, the need to support further development of IT capacity to manage patients remotely) and the general principles of good management and stewardship (for example, protecting the fabric of buildings for the longer term).

Another primary care manager noted the importance of a deep understanding of the strategic plan: 'The fundamental issue is the cohesion and strategic acumen of your board of gover-nance ... you have got to have a very diligent board which understands the mission of your organisation.'

There might be times when organisations do take on projects that do not fit clearly within their strategic directions and there might be good reasons for doing so. For example, you might want to explore a particular issue to see if it is something you should take up, or to develop a relationship with a particular group or funding body. If this is the case, it is vital to be clear about why you are doing it and what you will do if it does or does not work out.

2. *Does it fit with our culture and values, or what we want them to be—really?*

> 'Culture eats strategy for lunch.' (*Bard Group*)

We have emphasised the importance of aligning the project portfolio with the organisation's strategic directions, but we have also noted the difficulties human service organisations experience in moving in a coordinated way. Culture clash is a powerful source of some of these difficulties.

One of our informants expressed the problem of projects that clash with the culture in this way: 'They are conflicting with the current culture and therefore they don't get the support and they might have a bit of a start but they never really get going.' This demonstrates the waste involved in ignoring the 'feral' culture, the real working rules. We are not suggesting that such projects should never be attempted, but rather that the existence of such barriers must be identified and a method for dealing with them factored into the project plan—either pragmatically (through clever avoidance) or through effective change management strategies.

Another way of thinking about this is to consider the fact that many projects are focused on achieving improvement through changing the way operational processes work. Such projects occupy the 'white spaces in the organisation chart' (Rummler and Brache 1995); that is, they focus on processes in which typically several teams or departments are involved—as with the washing up, everyone and no one is in charge.

This is also the area where much of the feral culture of the organisation is created. For example, one hospital CEO reported on a project idea that aimed to 'do work redesign between doctors and nurses and allied health'. In spite of strong agreement at a strategic planning workshop, the hospital has not been able to do anything effective. The reasons given are that 'it is too hard and you need thinking time and people just can't come to terms with it'. This explanation has all the hallmarks of a problem of culture clash—in this case, the preference of members of a profession for working with each other rather than other groups.

Having emphasised the importance of specific goals as a guide to project selection, we are now suggesting that it is worthwhile to check the project fit with more general culture and values in two ways. First, does the project, its goals and methods, sit well with the values we aspire to? And second, will this project raise 'antibodies' because it cuts across some of the strongly held imperatives of the 'shadow side' of the organisation, the values or practices we wish were different?

If the answer to the second question is 'yes', then decisions must be made as to whether the project offers a good opportunity to challenge these values and practices, and how this might be done. The other option is to look for ways of circumnavigating the point where the clash of values occurs. It may be, however, that the culture problem is so strong that the project is doomed to failure and should not be taken on.

3. Is this a project or an elephant?

We have discussed the problem of woolly thinking about worthy goals—having a good idea, or a worthy aspiration, does not necessarily translate into a feasible project. Projects need both a goal and a practical method—they need to be clearly defined, concrete and achievable within a timeframe that can be reasonably estimated. Without a method, you may have a pressing problem or a great opportunity, but you will not have a project. The means of solving the given problem, or taking advantage of the opportunity, need to be clearly identified and available.

4. Is there a leader for this project, a sponsor who will make sure it delivers?

Lack of leadership was seen as a problem by several of our informants, at two levels. The first is the level of the project team (see Chapter 6), but here we are focusing on the second— someone in a leadership position who is prepared to sponsor or champion this project, to be the person who will provide influence and access to needed resources when the team needs it. 'Top management support' is often cited in the project management literature as a make-or-break factor (e.g. White and Fortune 2002), and our research supports this. But the level and type of support that is needed will vary widely depending on the project and the organisation's structure and style.

This issue was highlighted strongly by the government department staff we interviewed: 'If you haven't got high-level endorsement and championing it is very hard to make even a very good idea work.' Another person observed, 'Projects require individuals to have some passion about them. And if that individual goes, they can fall apart—I think it's surprisingly individually dependent.'

5. Does this project require partners, and if so, is this feasible?

Failure to recognise the external implications of projects is a common problem reported in the literature, including White and Fortune's large study (2002). Our informants spoke often of the need for effective partnerships to achieve many of the service development projects they had embarked upon. A GP division manager quoted a major project (with over $2 million in funding) which involved five other divisions: 'We learnt that you don't go down the pathway alone. If you want to do something really cutting edge, you must form a coalition.'

The challenge is to recognise the need for partnerships in the early stages and to manage them well. Organisations which are more engaged with their environments and their communities, and have established more robust relationships, are better placed both to see the implications and to move quickly to respond to them.

6. Do we have, or can we readily get, the skills to succeed with this project?

Again, we are not only referring to project management skills, but also to the core competencies of the organisation—are we innovators or implementers? Do we have the basic technological know-how to support this project and its results? Are we in a position to work well with the intended client group, and with the key funders and regulators?

This criterion can also be used for consideration of the human resource questions—will this project provide good opportunities for the development of project skills and for career development?

7. Can we handle the resource requirements in a timely manner?

This question is not simply about accurate estimation and securing the direct funding requirements of the project—these issues will be addressed in Part 2. The question here is about the capability of the organisation to mobilise the skills, staffing and management attention required to support effective project management. Case 4 gives a brief example.

Case 4: The killer resource problem

A primary care manager described a project which failed because of 'wilful blindness' to a fatal flaw. The project aimed to improve timely access to cardiology services through better coordination of care: 'We should have known before we even started there were never going to be enough cardiologists to do the work. There was a short supply of them and that is why we were trying to do it, we should have known that the short supply was going to shoot us in the foot.' She believed that the wilful blindness was the result of charismatic people carrying the day in the absence of sufficient 'spade work' or due diligence.

8. If it succeeds, are the results sustainable?

This was an important problem for most of the organisations we studied. As a community health service manager put it: 'It is no good piloting something if we then don't have the resources to integrate it into the organisation, so there has to be that ongoing capacity to maintain it.'

A manager in a large health service commented on 'the lack of accountability and the lack of follow through, so we are quite good at setting up things but we lack the discipline to actually come back and make sure that it is still going'.

9. Will this project contribute to our organisational learning and competence?

Related to the theme of sustainability is the question of the potential for projects to contribute to the development of the organisation, its core competencies and organisational learning. We argue that this learning and development potential should rank strongly as a criterion when the project portfolio is being compiled.

The checklist on page 54 summarises our analysis of project portfolio selection. It is necessarily generic—we suggest that individual organisations could refine the list to focus it more strongly on their unique considerations.

The checklist: which projects should we do?

1. Will this project help to achieve our *strategic goals*, directly or indirectly?
2. Does it fit with our *culture and values*, or what we want them to be—really?
3. Is it a *project* or an elephant?
4. Is there a *leader* for this project, a champion who will make sure it delivers?
5. Does this project require *partners*, and if so, is this feasible?
6. Do we have, or can we readily get, the *skills* to succeed with this project?
7. Can we handle the *resource requirements* in a timely manner?
8. If it succeeds, are the results *sustainable?*
9. Will this project contribute to our *organisational learning* and competence?

SUMMARY

- There are three key influences which enable or constrain project success across the sector. The first is proliferation of project funding programs, designed to promote innovation and improvement. The second is idealism and commitment to the public good, which leads staff to overestimate what is achievable and underestimate time and resource requirements. It also causes difficulties in prioritising among competing needs. The third is the existence of multiple empowered stakeholders with disseminated leadership and multiple agendas, which make it hard to establish strong agreed strategic directions and pursue them vigorously.

- Government departments are deeply involved in project work, and experience a clash between the project management approach and the complexities and vagaries of government and bureaucracy.

- Government offers significant funding for projects, but the timing and criteria are sometimes difficult for service delivery organisations to manage.

■ There are five key factors that underlie the capability of organisations to succeed in project management: strategic directions, leadership, organisation structure, a 'project management culture' and human resource management.
■ Human service organisations need a strategic approach to their project portfolios, including the selection of projects, and the management of project capacity.
■ The project portfolio checklist provides a set of criteria for selecting the projects which are likely to succeed and which contribute to organisational strategy and development.

This brings us to the conclusion of Part 1, in which we have addressed the 'big picture' in project management. Part 2 turns to the practical management of projects.

Part 2

MANAGING PROJECTS SUCCESSFULLY

In Part 2 we turn to the process of managing projects, and the requirements for success. The next five chapters provide an explanation of the language, frameworks, tools and methods that are commonly used in project management, and of how to select and adapt them to suit the project in hand and the organisation. This part of the book is structured according to the project life cycle. That is, we begin at the beginning—somebody has a good idea or a problem needing a solution—and work through to project completion and evaluation.

Through our research, and our reading of the literature, we identified four major requirements for project success, as outlined in the Model for Project Success Factors (see Figure 1, page 20):

- Commitment—a vision that supports the project, a willingness to do what is needed to make it work, and determination to see it all the way through.
- Plan and design—due diligence to ensure that the project concept is sound and feasible, and that the project, especially its aim, is well defined, followed by the development of a clear plan, detailed enough to provide a working road map for the project team, and a structure for making decisions during the project's life.

- Resourcing—adequate provision for both the material and human resource requirements of the project, and the organisational capacity to bring them all together.
- Project team performance—a skilled project manager, effectively managing change, using the right methods and tools, supported by good decision making and management of stakeholders.

The material in this part of the book is based on this analysis of success factors, and the chapters are designed as a resource for those who seek to enhance their skills and knowledge in practical project management, both in the field and as students.

3

UNDERSTANDING PROJECT MANAGEMENT

'Great things are not done by impulse, but by a series of small things brought together.' (*Vincent van Gogh*)

In this chapter we introduce the language and methods of project management, and provide information about helpful resources.

PROJECT MANAGEMENT LANGUAGE

Managers in human service organisations have been undertaking project management activities for many years, but may not have labelled their activities as projects nor have been aware that tailored methods are available. As noted earlier, implementing a pilot program or a new way of doing something is a project even though it might not have been conceived of in this way. The human services sector is an area where many new developments and initiatives have been successfully implemented in recent years. Many of the people involved, ourselves included, have in fact learnt by doing, that is, we have taken a rational planning approach to the implementation of something new and used our managerial skills to ensure that it gets done. In some ways, the technical terms used in project management (for example, 'work breakdown structure', 'project scope', 'deliverables') are simply alternative labels for the activities that managers do as part of their daily work— setting goals and targets, deciding on strategy and working out tasks and responsibilities.

Not all professional staff have had broader managerial training or experience, yet we found the practice of expecting competent professional staff to be able to 'just do it' in project management to be a common problem in the sector.

Perhaps the first difficulty in understanding project management is understanding the language. In the project management literature there are myriad acronyms—for example, PERT (Project Evaluation and Review Technique), WBS (Work Breakdown Structure), and terms like Gantt chart, 'close-out', 'go-live' —it seems that project management has a language all of its own. The use of project terminology can be confusing, as it is not necessarily used consistently, but there is no need to be intimidated by the terms used by project managers, IT companies or project management literature. Ultimately, project management is about defining, planning, monitoring and controlling projects to ensure their success.

PROJECT MANAGEMENT MODELS

Project managers often speak about 'models' and 'tools' of project management. Sometimes they give the impression that use of their favourite model or tool is the only way for the project to succeed. But in fact, both our research and the White and Fortune (2002) survey confirm that there are several models of project management in use in the sector, and that many organisations use their own in-house model or no set model at all. While certain principles and methods are necessary for project success in most instances, there is no one best model or tool, and no single recipe for success.

A project management model is basically a framework that can be useful to help conceptualise and understand what project management is, and how and when to use project management tools. Using the frameworks does not guarantee successful outcomes, nevertheless they can provide useful guides and signposts. There are several proprietary or branded project management products available and we review two of the more recognised ones below.

Project Management Body of Knowledge (PMBOK)

Published by the US-based Project Management Institute (PMI), *A Guide to the Project Management Body of Knowledge* (PMBOK Guide 2000) is a basic reference that encapsulates 'the sum of knowledge within the profession of project management' and is the 'world's de facto standard for the project management profession' (PMI 2002: 4). The PMBOK Guide package includes a source guide for project management books. The main purpose of the PMBOK Guide is to identify and describe project management knowledge and practices that are generally accepted to be valuable and useful in most projects. The project management knowledge areas described in PMBOK include project integration, scope, time, cost, quality, human resource, communications, risk and procurement management. Rather than being a recipe book for successful project management, this publication is an excellent resource explaining theories and principles of project management, project processes and phases, and relevant tools and techniques.

We have drawn on PMBOK throughout these chapters.

PRINCE® and PRINCE2®

PRINCE (PRojects IN Controlled Environments) is a structured set of components, techniques and processes designed for managing any type or size of project (CCTA 1997). Owned by the Central Computer and Telecommunications Agency (UK), the PRINCE method is a process-based model for the management of projects, and includes templates and tools that provide 'a framework whereby a bridge between a current state of affairs and a planned future state may be constructed' (CCTA 1997). The philosophy behind the PRINCE model is that although every project is technically unique, having a single, common and structured approach to project management avoids the need to devise a specific approach for each project.

PRINCE has been used successfully in a number of large and small human service organisations; it provides an overview of project management theory, and very practical methods for thinking about how the project fits into the organisation, how to go about planning and initiating the project, and managing the stages of the project. The PRINCE package also includes actual templates that can be used as is or adapted—for example, a project brief, quality plan, business case, communications plan, risk log and end project report.

PRINCE was among the most commonly used methods in White and Fortune's survey (2002) and has now been mandated by some departments of the UK government as the required method for describing the management of funded projects (Roberts and Ludvigsen 1998).

There are many other frameworks available in a multitude of textbooks and manuals on project management, but they vary in their relevance to the human services sector. Some interesting alternatives are used in fields like international development work—the 'logframe' matrix—and agriculture—Bennett's Hierarchy (Bennett et al 2001; available on *http://citnews.unl.edu/TOP/english/contentsf.html*)—which seem promising for use in health and community services. We give more detailed consideration to these and other methods in Chapters 5, 6 and 7.

See later in this chapter for a listing of textbooks we have found to be useful.

PROJECT MANAGEMENT TOOLS

A project management tool is a mechanism by which a project task is achieved. Common tools are Gantt and PERT charts and computerised project management tools such as Microsoft Project or Mac Project™. Tools like these are aids in the project management process, and it is valuable to understand what they are and how they might be useful. However, it is not essential to use them to make your project work—in fact, with very complex projects such an approach can create more problems than it solves.

Many organisations have developed their own forms and templates and implemented software to facilitate some project management processes, so it is useful to check what is available in the workplace. If this is not fruitful, it is worth looking a bit further afield, for while the principles of project management are understood in some sections of the health and community services industry, a vast amount of information about the tools and techniques of project management is available in other industries, especially for project managers in engineering or IT fields. It must be said, however, that some of the more technical methods of project management are limited in their usefulness due to the complexity of the health and community services environment.

Project management is not just applying a set of pre-existing tools to a management issue with the expectation that a project or program will then be successful. Project management is an art, not an algorithm, and requires knowing under what circumstances to use it and what aspects to use (Kliem et al. 1997:31). Many project management tools and techniques will be ineffective unless they are supported by strong management practices, including effective negotiation, communication, leadership, alliances and networks, change management and a supportive or enlightened organisational culture.

Methods and tools used in health and community services

Our research indicates that not many health organisations are using a standardised or 'off the shelf' project management method throughout the organisation, but rather a variety of project management methods, tools and processes, some of them locally developed. Some tools, forms and templates developed for other uses in the organisation—for example, a proforma for risk analysis or status reporting—can be applied to a project setting. Some government departments have adopted a specific project management method like PRINCE or PMBOK and use it as a framework, a set of guiding principles for project management.

Whether a model of project management is used can depend on the source of funding. If the project involves a tender process or a consultancy, some standardised methods used by government may be stipulated as part of the funding arrangement, including methods of contracting, tendering and procurement, and rules of probity.

The method or the tool

There is a difference between a project method and a tool. The *method* is the principle of the activity; and the *tool* is the mechanism by which it is achieved. For example, monitoring the project schedule is an important method of ensuring timeliness, and the Gantt chart is a useful tool for the task. It is easy to get carried away with an impressive array of tools, but it is important not to lose sight of the underlying method and to choose the correct tools for success.

Some authors and managers believe that there is a technique or tool to cover any project management situation. For example, Kliem et al. (1997) state that project management is all about tools, knowledge and techniques for leading, defining, planning, organising, controlling and closing a project. Others firmly believe that a good manager is also a good project manager, that project management is really a case of commonsense based on experience, and that special tools and techniques do not necessarily add value. Project management methods can also be seen as a hindrance because they are too mechanistic, or as being of limited value in dealing with health and community organisations because they were designed for other environments. The balance is probably somewhere in the middle, in that formal project management methods have their place and are of particular value in some projects, but cannot of themselves ensure project success.

Computerised project management tools and technologies

A number of existing technologies assist in the management of projects and enable project managers and team members access to networked software and systems. These technologies include videoconferencing, the Internet, GroupWare and network database management systems, an Intranet and the World Wide Web (Lientz and Rea 1998). Both voice mail and electronic mail are invaluable for collecting and disseminating project information, and calender/scheduling software makes for easier coordination of project meetings.

There is a wide range of project management software packages available to assist in the management of projects and also in the establishment of an organisation-wide project management information system. But again, there is more to project management than just using project management software—it does not manage the project for you. Lientz and Rea (1998:131–47) give a good account of issues in the management of project technology and developing a project management network strategy. They also devote a chapter in their book to the functions and uses of project management software, software evaluation criteria and software packages. Pitfalls in buying and using project management software include:

- The purchased software is never used.
- The software is used for limited functions; for example as a drawing tool, for timekeeping or budgeting, and is not fully utilised.

- Inappropriate or overly sophisticated software is purchased and is unwieldy and too large to be useful.
- The project manager gets too involved in the software, to the detriment of the project.

Microsoft Project is a commonly used project management product which enables the establishment of Gantt, PERT and critical path charts, milestones, project baselines, resource allocation and a work breakdown structure. Unfortunately, training in the software is sometimes the only training that would-be project managers receive. It is important, when evaluating project management software, to have a good idea of which tools would assist in the management of individual projects, and whether there is a need for a management system for multiple projects. Project management software, as with any other IT application, needs to be thoroughly evaluated in relation to the organisation's existing systems, software and project/s. The process of evaluation and implementation of project management software is a project in itself.

There is a multitude of project management software products available, some of them web based and downloadable free. A software directory for over 100 project management software products, provided on the website *www.project-management-software.org*, includes: Vertabase Pro™, Autotask™, VCS™, Tenrox Project Tracking™, FreeTaskManager™, Project.net™ and Project Insight™.

THE PROJECT LIFE CYCLE

Projects are usually divided up into several phases or stages to make the project more manageable, and sometimes because each phase has associated outputs or 'deliverables' (that is, tangible, verifiable work products) (PMI 2000). For example, a project which aims to acquire and implement a new information system for registering clients of a mental health service will have several phases, each marked by the handing over of a deliverable (functionality confirmation perhaps, or curriculum for staff training programs).

Defining project phases and their outputs also enables progressive decisions to be made about whether or not to progress to the next phase. In the example above, there would be a requirement for 'sign-off' (formal acceptance by the client or sponsor of the project) before the next stage could proceed. Many projects do not continue after the initial analysis or definition phases for a variety of reasons, including that they were found not to be feasible, or not able to be completed within timeframes required by the organisation's strategic plan. Collectively, the project phases are known as the project life cycle.

The number of phases and the activities or deliverables in each phase depend entirely on the project and the industry within which it is being carried out. It is usual to have around four or five phases (but there could be more) that might be divided thus:

- *Concept phase:* Includes feasibility or needs analysis. This is sometimes called the feasibility, analysis, transition, strategy, conception, proof of concept or discovery phase. This is the phase that basically works out what you want to do and whether you can do it.
- *Definition phase:* Includes the project planning and design activities, and is sometimes referred to as the demonstration and validation, first build or preclinical deployment phase. In this phase you know what you want to do and you have to decide how you are going to do it.
- *Implementation phase:* Also known as the production, second build, construction or development phase. This is the difficult bit—making it all happen.
- *Completion and evaluation phase:* May also be known as the turnover and start up, go-live, final or production and deployment phase. In some projects this is where the product, deliverable or outcome is put into practice to see if it works; in others the evaluation is carried out by asking whether the project has met its aims and objectives and stakeholder expectations, or whether it did what it set out to do and is sustainable.

All projects contain these basic steps. The steps might be called different things, and certain stages might contain a greater number of steps than others depending on the nature and size of the project.

A health promotion project might contain the following phases:

- *Analysis phase:* Rationale, community needs analysis, literature review, action research.
- *Definition phase:* Developing the plan, setting goals and objectives, defining tasks, timelines, resources, responsibilities and outcomes.
- *Implementation:* hiring new staff, training existing staff, procurement of equipment, preparing material, organising and conducting workshops, seminars and project activities.
- *Closure:* evaluation and review, often including a decision about whether to sustain the outcomes of the project as an ongoing part of the organisation's services or products.

Projects involving the purchase or implementation of information technology can have a more complex life cycle than other projects, but essentially use the same tools and techniques to achieve project success.

An IT project may involve the following phases:

- *Analysis phase:* May include research, project scope, budgeting, acquiring capital funds, authorisation, finding a sponsor, specification development (technical, functional), planning of tendering process (expressions of interest), RFT (Request for Tender), vendor demonstrations, tender evaluation, contract with vendor, implementation planning study (undertaken by vendor), project initiation, planning workshops and functional, technical document production.
- *Design phase:* May include design of project management structure, technical architecture, product delivery, data migration, integration, implementation strategy, development, training strategy, testing strategy, issues and risk management strategy.
- *Implementation phase:* Technical configuration, system configuration, system integration, system migration, software implementation, system testing (acceptance, user acceptance, regression), user training.
- *Go-live phase:* Go-live schedule, operational readiness testing, process data migration, fix any rejected data, go-live support.
- *Post implementation phase:* Transition from project status to support status, review outstanding issues, project review, closure.

This does not mean that the health promotion project is any less complex than an information technology project. The implementation phase of the health promotion project might require the staff to work differently and in different teams, and it may have many of the features of an organisation change project, hopefully identified and planned for before the project progressed too far.

These examples demonstrate the rational approach of the project lifecycle. This way of thinking about the stages of a project, however, can mask a whole series of practical problems and difficulties that can emerge, often when people are asked to do things differently. As we explore each of the major project activities and tasks, this issue of the rhetoric versus the reality of projects, and ways of dealing with the gaps between the rational approach and the 'shadow side' (Egan 1994) will be addressed.

PROJECT MANAGEMENT RESOURCES FOR MANAGERS

Finally in this chapter, we present a short guide to finding project management resources which can assist project staff to skill up quickly and assist students of project management to find their way around the literature. These resources, many of them available free in libraries and over the Internet, include project management text books, Internet sites, databases, journals, organisations and training courses.

Project management textbooks

A number of practical and useful project management textbooks are available, with varying amounts of jargon and technical complexity. There are not many texts that explore project management in the health industry, hence the need for this book. The following are suggested as good all-round project management texts that project managers (and students) might find useful when investigating project management theory or when initiating or managing a project:

- Billows, D. (2000) *Essentials of Project Management: Focus on using MS Project* (can be ordered at *http://www.4pm.com*)
- CCTA (1999) *PRINCE: An Outline*, The Stationery Office, London (difficult to obtain hard copy, go to Prince2 website— *http://www.prince2.com*)
- Healy, Patrick (1997) *Project Management: Getting the job done*

on time and on budget, Butterworth Heinemann, Sydney
- Lientz, B. and Rea, K. (1998) *Project Management for the 21st Century*, 2nd edition, Academic Press, San Diego
- Meredith, J. and Mantel, S. (2000) *Project Management: A managerial approach*, 4th edition, John Wiley & Sons, New York
- Roberts, K. and Ludvigsen, C. (1998) *Project Management for Health Care Professionals*, Butterworth Heinemann, Oxford
- Rosenau, M.D. (1998) *Successful Project Management: A step by step approach with practical examples*, John Wiley & Sons, New York
- Webster, Gordon (1999) *Managing Projects at Work*, Gower Publishing Limited, Hampshire

Project management journals

The *International Journal of Project Management* (based in the UK) and the *Project Management Journal* (published by the Project Management Institute, based in the USA) are the leading journals dedicated to project management theory and practice. Most professional and management journals also carry articles about project management in their specific areas from time to time.

Useful Internet sites and project management organisations

- The Australian Institute of Project Management, *www.aipm. com.au*—the peak body for project management in Australia
- The US-based Project Management Institute, *www.pmi.org*
- Project Management Forum, *www.pmforum.org*
- Association for Project Management, *www.apm.org.uk*—the UK peak body
- International Project Management Association, *www.ipma.ch*—based in Europe
- The Project Management Centre, *www.infogoal.com/pmc/pmchome.htm*—the PMC brings together project management information on software, seminars, training, articles, books, news, links, organisations, standards and project management job opportunities
- *www.gantthead.com* a fun site directed primarily to IT project managers.
- Enhanced Management Framework, *IT Project Managers Handbook*. Provides an online project management model and handbook directed to large scale public sector projects, *www.cio-dpi.gc.ca/emf-cag*

Project management seminars, courses, careers and professional development

A number of organisations offer courses, training and professional development in project management, including universities, project management organisations, consulting firms, higher and adult education facilities and registered training organisations. Project management education is available by distance education, online, on site and face to face; however, very little of what is on offer is tailored to projects or project managers in the health and community services sector. There is no single recognised qualification in project management in the sector, mainly due to the wide range of projects undertaken and the fact that the majority of project managers gain project management skills and experience on the job. The following training programs are not necessarily recommended or endorsed by the authors, but are suggestions only. Alternatively, scan your local university and further education websites for courses on project management:

- Online seminars in project management and managing multiple projects, available at *www.learningstream.com*
- Online Certificates in Project Management offered by Villanova University (Pennsylvania USA), at *www.VillanovaU.com*
- UNE Partnerships Pty Ltd (the education and training company of the University of New England, Armidale, New South Wales, Australia) offers a Diploma, Advanced Diploma and Certificate IV in Project Management by Distance Education; more information at *www.unepartnerships.com*
- Melbourne University Private, School of Enterprise offers short courses, consultancies and professional development in the area of project management; see *www.muprivate.edu.au/schools/soe*

PROJECT MANAGEMENT CAREERS

In the wider health industry there is evidence of increasing demand for project managers and project officers. A quick scan of the newspaper shows that there are many opportunities at all levels and sectors of the health industry for fixed-term project positions for those with health industry experience and qualifications. Contract and project-based employment arrangements increasingly suit employers in the current funding environment.

Case 5: Recruiting project staff

These are two examples of advertisements for project staff.

Project Manager—Hospital Based
Full time, fixed term for three years

Coordinated Healthcare is seeking an enthusiastic person to join their team, in the role of Project Manager. The Project Manager will be responsible for managing projects relating to the Coordinated Healthcare Trial, managing project staff, ensuring that project objectives are met, while also assisting in the coordination of operations, to ensure the timely achievement of Commonwealth and Health Service goals for all project activities.

The successful candidate will have experience in project management, previous health sector experience or qualifications and demonstrate high-level communication skills, both oral and written.

Project Officer—Nurse Education
Policy & Strategic Projects/Nurse Policy

The Nurse Policy Branch is seeking a suitably experienced person to fulfil the role of Project Officer—Education. The position is responsible to Manager, Nursing Policy for advice, comment and policy development on nurse education issues.

Applicants will need to possess good writing and analytical skills and have excellent understanding of undergraduate, postgraduate and continuing nursing education issues. It is essential they have a good understanding of the sector.

There is also an emerging career structure for project managers. Larger organisations are appointing senior project managers to positions which require them to plan, acquire funding and coordinate a set of major projects. Sometimes the leader of the project effort is also the senior planning and development officer for the organisation and a member of the executive. Experienced health project managers are also recruited by consulting firms to jobs which offer increasingly complex project management tasks and team leadership and management roles.

SUMMARY

- Project management has a unique language, but many of the principles are familiar to experienced managers.
- There are a number of project management frameworks, models and tools that assist in understanding project management concepts and theories; however, no single approach or method can guarantee project success.
- The Project Management Body of Knowledge and PRINCE2 are sound and useful frameworks for managing projects.
- Project management software can be useful, and there are many good products available, but they do not substitute for leadership and sound management.
- An understanding of the principles and theories of project management is important for the project manager in health and community services; however, as in general management there is no one best way and project managers need to use their own judgment and discretion.
- There are many valuable resources available to assist project managers, including books, Internet sites, journals, seminars and courses.
- There are increasing opportunities and an emerging career structure for project managers in health and community services.

4

THE CONCEPT PHASE:
WHAT DO YOU WANT TO DO
AND WHY?

'From little things big things grow.' (*Paul Kelly*)

This chapter introduces the first stage of the project life cycle—turning good ideas into practical project proposals for implementation. We first of all ask 'Where do ideas for projects come from?' and then consider the methods of turning good ideas into projects. We include a number of established tools and models for developing and testing ideas in health and community services specifically, and address the question of how to get support for your project ideas. The chapter concludes with a discussion of funding for projects, responding to tendered projects or funding rounds, and contracting projects to consultants.

WHERE DO IDEAS COME FROM?

'Good ideas for projects come from anywhere.' (*GP division manager*)

Projects generally emerge from the combination of an organisational need—to solve a problem or take up an opportunity—and a good idea about how to meet that need. In our research we found that indeed good ideas for projects arose everywhere, and that the process of emergence and capture of good ideas varies with the size and nature of the organisation and its approach to innovation and development. For example, in large organisations it is often the leadership group which identifies problems that need a project-based solution and commissions project work. This top-down approach has the advantage of senior management support and therefore better access to resources. However, if the project requires change in the processes of service delivery, it may be more difficult to get staff further down the hierarchy to own and support it (this support is known in project management language as 'buy in').

Sometimes projects emerge from a change in the law; for example a new occupational health and safety requirement, or because someone thinks of a better way of doing something and lobbies decision makers to test it out. Problems that need solutions might emerge in team meetings or during informal discussions between staff, and be developed into project ideas. Other management activities, such as organisational needs analysis, might give rise to a series of projects designed to enhance staff or system performance.

Good ideas then depend on funding opportunities, organisational strategic directions, individual passion and sometimes serendipity, in order to survive and be developed into potential projects. The use of formal project 'rounds' was quite widespread among our informants, with several different characteristics. One large hospital reported increasingly disciplined use of the three-yearly strategic planning process as the primary agenda-setting mechanism, with an annual round for internally-funded projects based on that agenda. In this organisation, the importance of sticking to the plan was becoming accepted, and groups within the organisation knew that they needed to focus on input to the strategic plan in order to advance their own agendas. The plan was also used as the basis for determining support for external funding bids.

The development of open, participative processes for determining the priority for submissions for external funding was also a common theme—see Case 6.

'Good ideas sheets' (see Figure 2) are sometimes used to assist in the development of new project or program ideas as part of a wider process for discussion and approval to move from ideas to plans. The value of such an approach is that staff are encouraged to articulate their ideas and think them through if

Case 6: Using participation to develop project ideas

One large health service reported on its response to a funding program which had very clear objectives and addressed an issue that was a high priority for the organisation. The whole organisation was asked to identify potential projects or initiatives using a brief proforma designed to collect good ideas while minimising the burden of writing the initial proposals. About 300 submissions were received.

A workshop with over 50 participants, including consumers and other external stakeholders, went through a process of bringing the 300 down to 12, with a great deal of grouping and melding of ideas through discussion. A 'village marketplace' was created through which people were able to add value or combine ideas, with ultimate prioritising through 'dotmocracy' (voting by allocation of coloured dots) so all 50 people voted. The organisation's executive then endorsed the top 12 for submission.

While this process consumed a lot of energy, it generated a set of ideas that were well tested and broadly supported, with an overt, transparent process. The manager believed that the process was worth it for the organisation for several reasons, one being the need to ensure broad support for the projects that were ultimately implemented.

they want to get support, and that ideas can be assessed early on for fit with the strategic directions of the organisation.

MOVING BEYOND WORTHY GOALS

One of the fundamentals of project management is the principle that you first decide *what* you want to achieve, then work out specifically *how* to do it. There is of course an interaction between the 'what' and the 'how'—people always tailor their goals according to their means as well as finding the means to achieve their goals. But the principle remains, and the staging of project development accordingly is important: be clear about what you want to do, agree on how you're going to do it and then get on with it.

Figure 2: Creative ideas sheet

Creative Ideas Sheet

This form is designed to support the bringing of good ideas into practice. It should be completed and approved as the first phase in the development of new projects or programs.

The next phase is development of a project/program proposal, which is ultimately approved by the management team.

Step 1: Outline a good idea

Step 2: Discuss with site manager

Step 3: Present idea in detail to site staff meeting for discussion

Name/s ....

....

Site:

Creative idea (please describe here and append one page only if necessary)

Discussed with site manager   Supported   Y/N   Date:

Discussed with site team   Supported   Y/N   Date:

Discussed at Management Team meeting   Supported   Y/N   Date:

Project/program proposal to be completed by: Date:

Source: Adapted from Peninsula Community Health Service, Victoria

We use the terms 'aim' and 'goal' to mean the same thing, that is, what it is that you intend your project to do. What do you want to achieve? Clarity is essential, whether you want to establish a support group for carers of children with disabilities, introduce a new model of care for stroke sufferers, develop a new occupational health and safety program, establish a service for newly arrived African women migrants, reduce the risk of positive lab results not being acted on or enable home nurses to record and retrieve data from their cars.

This may seem so obvious as not to need such emphatic statement. But our experience in teaching, research and practice has taught us that one of the most challenging tasks in developing a project is defining the goal in a way that lends itself to implementation and achievement. In health and community services people often have a passion for doing good and the energy and commitment to do it, but if they are not clear exactly what they are aiming for when they begin, the project is in trouble from the start. The classical project management literature also stresses poor definition of what the project is trying to achieve as a factor in project failure (PMI 2000:57), and the people we interviewed emphasised over-ambitious goals as a big issue, in that people seem to naturally overestimate what they can do. Case 7 illustrates the value of project definitions.

Case 7: From aspiration to project goal

Staff in a small community agency were interested in reducing tobacco smoking in young women, and they felt that this should be their project goal. After some investigation and some hard thinking about the resources at their disposal, they recognised that such a goal was not achievable, and did not enable them to define clear indicators of success. They defined a project which involved working with the peak tobacco control body, and the schools in their community, to ensure that young women in their area had access to skilled support during a major citywide campaign on smoking based on television advertisements and a computerised information package. Their new goal was 'to ensure that young women in our community have access to skilled support for reducing tobacco use through their schools and teachers'.

> They had not let go of their aspiration to contribute to reducing the health consequences of smoking, but they had committed to a focused, achievable goal—the first building block of a successful project.

In the early stages of a project it can be very difficult to take the step of turning a worthy aspiration into an achievable project goal, for many reasons. Sometimes it is simply lack of familiarity with the particular technical meaning of goals in project management, but it may also be due to conflicting priorities among staff designing the project, or to problems in matching the team's goals to the requirements of the funding agency. Whatever the reason, the process of getting to a focused goal almost always forces greater clarity about methods, timelines and the meaning of success. Now is the time, at the concept stage, to debate the need for the project, the evidence for effective responses, the project's relevance to the agency or unit's strategic goals, and the potential to gain allies and support. At this stage, debate about these issues can be enormously productive. Later on, when resources have been committed and movement towards the goal has begun, such debate can cripple a project's chance of success.

TURNING IDEAS INTO PROJECTS

Many projects begin as a vision held by one or two people, who then face the challenge of getting their initial idea to the stage of being recognised as a project, developed and approved for implementation. The other major pathway in health and community services is that an invitation to submit proposals for funding is received—from either internal or external sources—and good ideas are stimulated or pulled from bottom drawers and dusted off in response.

Turning vague concepts into achievable projects is the first task of project development. The creative ideas sheet (see Figure 2) can be used to test the project idea against established criteria (including the extent to which the proposed project fits with the organisation's strategic plan) and this constitutes the first stage of project definition and approval. Approval by the organisation then establishes sufficient support to enable the next stage of development.

A 'project proposal', 'project brief', 'project scope' or 'project definition' document is another useful tool for moving from a good idea to a defined project. Some organisations use templates or proformas to ensure that project proposals address all the major issues in a standard format. This is common practice in consulting firms, but was not widely used among the organisations we surveyed. Like any tool, project templates can become bureaucratic impediments if they are poorly designed or inappropriately used. Well-designed templates can be a valuable way of guarding against woolly thinking, as they assist proponents to identify whether their vision or good idea can really be translated into practical action by the organisation or team.

The project proposal template in Figure 3, adapted from one of the organisations we surveyed, is designed to prompt proponents to think through the precise goals and deliverables, the required resources, the costs and benefits, the support from key stakeholders and the major components of work that will be required to get the project to successful completion.

Template documents can vary widely depending upon the nature and type of the project and the organisation. The high-level project proposal format illustrated in Figure 3 can be used by project initiators to briefly document and discuss their ideas (in 2–3 pages maximum), prior to any formal authorisation process. This tool can also be used by senior management to get an overview of what projects are being initiated within the organisation, to enable the monitoring and management of the organisation's project portfolio.

In the next sections we present three established planning and decision-making methods which can also be useful at this stage of project development, or which with luck might have already been used to provide useful input to your project defi-nition. Needs analysis, economic evaluation and literature reviews (to establish the base of evidence) are not essential steps in project development, but rather are related methods which add value to projects in health and community services at the concept stage.

Needs analysis and priority setting

Any project plan should have a rationale—in other words, Why are you doing this? On what evidence do you think there is a

Figure 3: Project proposal template

Name of project:

Project sponsor: **Proposer:**

1. **Background to the project:** (Briefly explain what event led the project idea to arise)

2. **Goals and objectives:** (What is the project aiming to achieve?)

3. **Rationale:** (Why should these goals be pursued through a project?)

4. **Broad scope of the project:** (Briefly state the boundaries of the project, i.e. what is included and what is excluded?)

5. **Deliverables:** (What will this project produce?)

6. **Stakeholders:** (Who has power and influence, or a material stake, in this project? What are their concerns likely to be?)

7. **Timeframe and resourcing estimates?** (What is the likely duration of the project? Likely types and amounts of resources (labour and non labour) required? What is the likely source of funding?)

8. **Risks and key assumptions:** (Identify all known major risks the project faces, and outline the major assumptions made in this proposal)

Signoff:
Proposer: Sponsor:
Date: Date:

need? If the reason for your project is to respond to a particular health problem or community need, a thorough needs assessment, to establish exactly what the problem is, and whether or not the proposed program or project is the best response to it, may be an essential early step. Unfortunately, all too often projects are commissioned that, while they may be brilliantly conceived and even executed, are not related to an identified need.

Case 8: Developing a municipal public health plan (MPHP)

In the mid-1990s the Healthy Cities and Shires Project in Queensland developed a Municipal Public Health Planning (MPHP) project that was based on a participatory approach to health planning (Chapman and Davey 1997). The process had seven stages. The first—doing the groundwork—involved awareness raising and gaining commitment from key stakeholders. In order to do this a feasibility study was undertaken to assess the potential for the introduction of a local MPHP. A feasibility study is a form of exploratory research or small-scale pilot study often carried out when you are unsure as to whether what you have in mind 'has legs'.

The next stage built on the findings and experience gained in the feasibility study and clarified the way in which the project was to be managed. Working within guiding principles of collaboration and participation, all projects within the bigger project set up intersectoral committees. Establishing the roles and ground rules for these committees became important issues, for example, whether they were steering groups (which implies an element of control) or advisory groups (which suggests a different role). There was a great deal of sensitive negotiation between key stakeholders at this stage.

The third stage was a needs assessment with three components. The first component was the community profile that identified the specific demographic and health-related issues and risk factors in the local community, for example, age, income, gender and ethnicity. This component also included a review of relevant previous research into indicators of need in the local area. The second component was an internal analysis which drew on the feasibility study and enabled the project team to assess whether the local organisation involved was ready to implement an MPHP. The third component was a community consultation process which explored what the community thought their health needs were. Priority issues were determined, followed by the development of strategies and the writing of the draft plan. The final stage was monitoring, review and evaluation of the MPHP.

The needs assessment outlined in Case 8 resulted in a large amount of information, most of it very valuable, but the teams experienced some difficulty in limiting the scope of the needs assessment. Another difficulty in community needs assessments of this kind lies in raising false hopes or identifying issues and problems that are well beyond the scope of the organisation carrying out the project. Chapman and Davey (1997:89) argue that a participatory approach to health planning requires 'persistence, flexibility and a belief in the process'. Their analysis demonstrates the challenges of involving the community in a planning process but also the benefits for the community and the key stakeholders that result from such involvement.

Establishing priority needs should be part of an agency's regular long-range planning, but needs should be checked from time to time to ensure that organisational programs and projects continue to meet those priority needs and that programs and projects are contributing to achievement of the organisation's basic purpose.

In analysing community needs these questions are often considered:

- How prevalent is the problem—how many people experience it?
- How severe is it—does it cause serious debilitation or minor inconvenience?
- Does the problem affect a particular group, especially a group that is disadvantaged in other ways?
- Are there known effective interventions that the program could promote and introduce? (Hawe et al. 1990)
- What are the costs and benefits of this particular project?

(This refers not only to the dollar costs, but also to the intangible costs and benefits such as opportunity costs—the value of opportunities forgone—or the benefit of health or welfare gain in a community.)

Organisations also do needs assessments for internal purposes, such as analysing the need for a human resource development program (DeSimone et al. 2002:128). The needs identified through such a process may lead to training and staff development activities, but they typically also identify other types of needs; for example, to overhaul the way work is done, the way jobs are structured or the arrangements for staff car parking. Any of these identified needs might require the development and implementation of a project. And if so, the detailed data gathered as part of the needs assessment will be a vital input to the project definition.

Economic evaluation

Cost benefit analysis, cost effectiveness analysis and cost utility analysis are techniques used in economic evaluation of interventions or services. Cost benefit analysis estimates the costs and benefits of a given intervention compared with another intervention, and identifies a dollar figure. In recent years, cost benefit analysis has been criticised precisely because it reduces complex values, such as quality of life, to a dollar figure.

Cost effectiveness analysis (CEA) and cost utility analysis (CUA) are more finely tuned forms of economic evaluation that express outcomes in non-monetary terms. CEA uses 'natural units' such as cure rate or reduction in the incidence of a disease; CUA attempts to express outcomes in quality adjusted life years (QALYs) so that comparisons of benefit can be made across diseases or conditions.

Economic evaluation is normally carried out by health or welfare economists, who assume that resources are scarce and see economic evaluation as an aid to rational allocation of resources. Concepts such as opportunity cost (achieving one sort of benefit at the expense of other benefits) and marginal analysis (making decisions on the relationship between the last dollar spent on a program or intervention and the benefit received for that dollar, rather than focusing on the average benefit of the program) are used. Economic evaluation 'in theory allows decision makers to be more rational in determining which projects to fund or expand and which to cut or contract' (Carter and Harris 1999:154).

Two useful basic texts on economic evaluation in health and community services are Gold et al. (1996), *Cost Effectiveness in Health and Medicine,* a US perspective on economic evaluation of health care formulated for the US national public health service, and Drummond et al. (1997), *Methods for the Economic Evaluation of Health Care Programmes,* the standard UK reference.

Using the evidence: literature reviews

Literature reviews are becoming increasingly common practice in the health and community services sector, and can be a valuable step in the development of projects. Literature reviews are mandatory in most academic research disciplines, but have become more widespread in recent years as part of important developments in medicine, in quality management and the eternal search for efficiency.

The principle of 'evidence-based medicine' or 'evidence-based healthcare' (Muir Gray 1997), now often expanded to 'evidence-based practice', is that decisions about treatments or interventions should be based on an objective evaluation of the best available evidence of effectiveness. The concept of 'best practice', on the other hand, arose in industry, and focuses on a comparison of current methods and outcomes in your company or agency with those of the best in your field, and then emulating their approaches. These ideas were born as part of new methods for pursuing both quality and efficiency (or competitiveness in the case of best practice) in the late twentieth century. Literature reviews play an important role in both.

A literature review can be an effective way of defining a problem, finding the current thinking on a subject or assembling the evidence of effectiveness for an intervention or service. It can also prevent the problem of well-intentioned but ultimately harmful projects or programs that adversely affect the very groups they were targeted to assist.

'Warning to schools on "misguided" anti-suicide programs'
Some school suicide-prevention programs are doing more harm than good ... Poorly researched programs posed 'a very real danger' to vulnerable students ... There are a lot of prevention programs run by well-intentioned but misguided community-based groups ... *The Age* 8/3/03

Literature reviews can assist agencies to avert misguided or even harmful projects that fail because they either do not meet a need or suffer from serious technical flaws in the way they are carried out. In other words, literature reviews can provide the evidence for decision making as to whether and how a project should proceed.

Carrying out a literature review

A literature review is not a list of everything that has ever been written on the subject; rather it is a clear logical analysis of what is known, setting out the problem that is to be examined in a defined context. A literature review is usually carried out to provide clarity and focus to a research problem as well as to improve the research methodology and knowledge base (Kumar 1996:26). In project management, a literature review can help clarify woolly thinking and help project managers to move from a general idea to a specific goal by finding out what others have done and learnt and what is still to be done.

Searching the literature

The first stage in a literature review is finding the material, and this requires knowing what you are looking for, and defining your subject area. Librarians use the Library of Congress Subject Headings when they are cataloguing books; these subject headings can be useful to help you decide where to focus your search. Using them, you can search library catalogues to find useful books, reports and journals, and get a good idea of the range of material available. The downside is that you will probably unearth a huge amount of material, much of it irrelevant and possibly out of date, as books in particular age quickly. Also, government reports, while essential for understanding directions and policy etc. often present only the one viewpoint and can put a positive spin on activities and results that might be disputed in a more rigorous analysis.

There are also citation indexes such as the Social Science Citation Index, and indexes of journals that your librarian can help you with. These can help you track down valuable journal articles and abstracts that might not appear in the main catalogue. However, perhaps the easiest and most efficient way of carrying out a literature search is to use electronic sources. These include the electronic databases for journal articles. Here keywords are more valuable than general subject headings; most databases will have their own lists of keywords to help you search. Some valuable databases include: ABI Inform, Econlit, Proquest, Emerald for business and management and CINAHL and Medline for health-related papers.

The useful things about journal articles and academic papers are that they are often more up to date than books, and are subject to a peer review process intended to ensure some intellectual rigour. Research papers generally report on something that has been done, a discrete research project that has clear aims and objectives, methods and analysis of results. The difficulty with journal articles is that sometimes they too are reporting on material that is a few years old; they can also be very technical and difficult to read and understand.

Other valuable sources of information that can be accessed electronically are newspaper articles and websites. Both these sources can be problematic in that they are largely not subjected to review before publication, and can be biased, or driven by a desire to sell rather than inform. Their integrity needs to be checked.

Another approach to a literature search that is often ignored is the rather old-fashioned strategy of physically browsing through the library shelves. It is surprising what you will unearth on one of these treks, including reports and journals that you have never heard of and very up-to-date papers that have not yet appeared in any electronic citation.

Finally, the thing to remember in literature searching is the importance of organisation—in other words, taking notes, keeping records (not only of the source but also details like page numbers for easy reference later), highlighting important concepts and capturing interesting ideas and potentially useful quotes. There are several software programs (for example, Endnote™) designed to make it easier to record and cite references.

Making sense of what you find

When you start on a literature search you will unearth many references and sources well beyond the scope of what you are doing. Some will be obvious when you read the abstract and you will go no further, others you will have to read through to find whether they address your issue. The next stage is to tell the story of what you find. Researchers would see this as developing the theoretical framework and departure point for research activity—basing what you do on explicit theories and knowledge. In a project it involves setting the parameters of what you are doing and establishing what is known to provide a guide or a focus for planning and management. The literature review should tell the story that you want to tell and present your argument as to why your project is essential and/or valuable, and why it should be approached in a particular way.

If you want to know more about doing literature reviews, these two texts are useful sources: Hart (1998), *Doing a Literature Review: Releasing the Social Science Research Imagination*, and Polgar and Thomas (2000), *Introduction to Research in the Health Sciences*.

Not all ideas for projects need to emerge from, or be subjected to, the rigorous processes outlined above, which are of course costly and time consuming in themselves. Many other analytical techniques which may be helpful in the concept phase of project development may be found in the resources listed in Chapter 3, and in the quality management literature.

GETTING SUPPORT FOR YOUR PROJECT IDEAS

Managers and staff often express frustration about failing to win senior support for good ideas aimed at addressing problems in their areas of responsibility, or at taking advantage of opportunities to improve their work processes. We asked the managers in our study to tell us why projects did not get support in their organisations. Common reasons that the project did not address core business or did not fit in with strategic directions, was beyond the scope of the organisation or perhaps could only be supported if some other agency had a lead role. Perhaps the project was seen to be high risk or the personalities involved did not inspire confidence, particularly if there was no champion or the proponents were seen to lack leadership skills.

Turning the question around to ask 'How can I be more successful in getting support for my projects?' we suggest the following, based on the criteria for choosing projects presented in Chapter 2, especially if your organisation has not developed its own clear criteria:

■ Relate the project to achievement of *strategic goals*, directly or indirectly.

- Demonstrate (or imply) *good fit with culture* and values, existing and desired.
- Develop a *practical project plan.*
- Explain the need for a *sponsor* (and the rewards) and your confidence in your boss in this role.
- Deal with any *alliances or partnerships* that might be needed.
- Demonstrate that needed *skills* are available (or can easily be acquired).
- Make sure the *resource requirements* are manageable and well timed.
- Explain how the *results will be sustained.*
- Demonstrate how this project will contribute to *organisational learning* and competence.

Funding

We turn now to the question of funding, which affects almost all projects. Sometimes the potential financial benefit of a project is so clear that a decision to invest can be made on the basis of a positive 'business case' (Brody 2000). A business case is essentially a project plan and financial analysis which quantifies and schedules the costs of a project and the direct cost savings or increased revenue arising from the project—a positive business case is one in which the benefits outweigh the costs. IT projects are typically required to show a positive business case; equally typically, the returns are either smaller than claimed, or accrue later than planned.

Projects in the health and community services sector often cannot demonstrate a positive business case. While this might mean that they cannot be pursued without additional funding, it does not necessarily mean they lack merit. Perhaps they do not aim either to save costs or increase revenues, or perhaps the cost savings accrue elsewhere, or the benefits do not translate into increased revenue because of the nature of funding restrictions. Case 9 illustrates this point.

Even where projects have a positive business case, or where internal resources are available, it is possible that without external funding they will not happen. Seeking and securing funding is a skill in itself. There are an increasing number of sources of grant funding for projects for health and community

Case 9: Positive health outcomes: negative business case

A children's hospital identified that many young parents were unaware of the dangers of shaking babies (in a misguided effort to make them stop crying). Using donated funds, they undertook a major campaign, with an educational video and other resources. After a year they were able to demonstrate a dramatic reduction in the incidence of shaking, and the admission of babies with the resulting brain injuries. Because of technical aspects of the hospital's funding, revenue was potentially reduced rather than enhanced by this outcome. No positive business case for this intervention could be presented, but the merit of the project is obvious.

service agencies, each with different criteria and requiring different approaches. Rubin and Rubin (1992) suggest that while there is no sure-fire way of writing a project proposal that will be funded, the following should be included:

- Preface the proposal with a brief overview of the project's goals, budget and procedure for evaluation.
- Discuss the objectives of the project and the plans for achieving those objectives, and include evidence of the 'problem' and the project's solution to those problems.
- Describe the organisation (or department), its membership, what it has accomplished, and who has benefited. Relate any experience with the problem at hand.
- Explain precisely how the requested resources will be used by including a detailed project budget.
- Describe how the organisation will evaluate the success or failure of the project.

In praise of opportunism

We have focused in this chapter on the need for organisations and individuals to ensure that their project ideas are tested for feasibility and relevance to strategic directions, and have advocated creative thinking and careful choices. But the people we interviewed reminded us that there is also a place for opportunism, for several reasons. Sometimes an organisation needs to get runs on the board or build capacity: 'At times it is very hard to manage because you can't always get the money you want for the strategic priorities and directions. And you have to have a record of successful externally funded project management so it's a bit of a balance.' Another informant noted: 'The more you're getting in, the more you've got the opportunity to attract more and you're building up your profile.'

Governments also respond to political issues, which may create opportunities. For example, if media attention is drawn to a problem that becomes a burning community issue—such as the use of drugs or inhalants by teenagers—governments will often respond by setting up a task force or establishing a project funding line to do something about it.

SIGN-OFF

After doing the necessary research and gathering support for your project idea, there is a final step at the end of the concept phase, that of getting 'sign-off'. Sign-off means getting the formal go-ahead from all the major players to proceed to the next stage of the project, which is the planning phase. Not all projects will require formal signatories to the project proposal; however, it is always a good idea to get at least verbal agreement from the relevant authority prior to launching into the next phase.

RESPONDING TO TENDERS

Finally in this chapter, we address the question of responding to tenders or deciding to tender out a project. A tender is an offer submitted by interested bidders (organisations which apply or 'bid' to win the contract) to the agency commissioning the project (sometimes called the 'purchaser'), usually in response to a 'Request for Tender'(RFT), also known as an 'Expression of Interest' (EOI) or 'Call for Tender' (CFT). Some governments have promoted the 'competitive tendering' process in many industries, including the health sector, in order to get competitive pricing for the provision of services, and hence there are many opportunities for organisations to bid for and win contracts, often for ongoing service delivery, but also for projects. Government RFTs are advertised widely, both in the news media and on government websites, along with information about tendering policies and guidelines (for example, for information on competitive tendering and contracting, see *www.finance.gov.au/ctc*).

There are two distinct reasons for responding to a tender. The first is when a problem or a good idea has been considered for a long time and suddenly there is an opportunity to get some funding for it or a variation of it. The other scenario is a more opportunistic one: a tender appears for something that has not been previously considered, or is perhaps not part of the agency's strategic directions but seems to bring other opportunities, so a bid is made.

The questions and tips below are designed to help with the process of deciding whether to respond to a tender:

- Who is commissioning this project and why? Do you know what they are looking for?
- Do your homework, use networks and contacts to find out as much background as possible.
- Always read the project brief/tender specification or funding guidelines carefully and always follow the instructions.
- Remember the project is for them, not for you—answer every question and tell them what they want to hear.
- Are you trying to fit one of your projects into someone else's project? If so, it might be difficult to achieve your aims (or even put in a successful bid).
- Is the tender bid realistic in terms of time and cost?
- Do you have the necessary skills to carry out this project?
- Are the roles and responsibilities clear?
- Do you have the support of senior management?
- Will you generate new intellectual property (IP) or use your existing IP, and if so, can your IP rights be protected? (Government contracts can be fierce on this point.)

Remember the organisation that has tendered out this project has done so for a reason—which was not to give you the opportunity to finance one of your pet ideas.

OFFERING PROJECT TENDERS

For some organisations, projects mean involving consultants, so that as soon as a project has been identified it tends to go to outside consultants, either through a tendering process or because of the successful track record of a particular company.

Deciding to tender out a project can also be a tricky decision given the resources that are usually involved in preparing the specifications and the tender process itself. Before putting out a project for tender, it may be useful to consider the following:

- Why is there a need to tender out this project? Is it because it is cheaper, is there a lack of skilled staff, or is it a complex problem best solved by an independent outsider with specific technical expertise?
- Exactly what are the required goals and outcomes?
- How long is it expected it to take?
- What will happen if it takes longer?
- How much should it cost?
- Are there any hidden costs to the organisation that have not been budgeted for?
- Are the required roles, responsibilities, accountability and monitoring methods clearly described?
- How will this project be evaluated?
- What kinds of people are needed to carry out this project?
- Is there an allowance for the costs of contract management, and of responding to the consultants' needs for information and access to staff?
- Are the skills and resources needed to manage the contract well available?
- Have any IP issues been identified and can they be resolved satisfactorily?

Essentially the tender process involves a number of steps, all necessary to ensure the best possible outcome and to fulfil the organisation's obligation to treat all bidders fairly. Key steps include:

1. The development of specifications for the project.
2. Preparing a Request for Tender (RFT) document.
3. Calling for expressions of interest and tenders.
4. Receipt and evaluation of tenderers' submissions.
5. Process for responding to queries and other contacts with tenders.
6. Notifying successful and unsuccessful bidders.

7. Contract negotiations.
8. Signing the contract.

Public organisations are usually expected to advertise tenders over a specified dollar amount; usually they are advertised in newspapers. The tender process must follow the principles of probity (the integrity of the tender process), which include fairness, impartiality, transparency, security, confidentiality and compliance with legislative obligations and government policy.

The discipline imposed by the tendering process can be helpful in forcing clear specification and sticking to the project plan. However, it can also cause problems when genuine contingencies arise and specifications, or methods and timelines need to be changed.

We'll give the final word on this topic to one of our informants, who took a strong position on the resources needed to manage a contracted project: 'I've got a rule in my head that says that for every consultant you bring into a project, you have to apply equal resources inside the project, because the consultancy is only as valuable as the internal working. The intellectual ownership and grunt has got to be internal, not external.'

Summary

- Ideas for projects originate from both within and outside the organisation, with many instigated by government and other funders.
- Within an organisation, ideas for projects can be captured, evaluated and progressed using both formal and informal processes; for example, by using an 'ideas sheet' or a project proposal document.
- A project must have clear, achievable aims.
- The project concept phase may involve performing the relevant background work or research, including needs analysis, economic evaluation or literature review, to ensure that the need for the project is established, that the evidence on how to design the project is gathered and that the project can meet its aims and objectives.
- To get a project from idea to implementation requires getting support and funding and may require sign-off before moving to the planning stage.

- Projects may involve responding to a request for tender or tendering to bring in consultants. These processes require strong planning and impose tight discipline on a project, which may be helpful by encouraging everyone to stick to the plan, or problematic when genuine contingencies emerge.

5

THE PLANNING PHASE:
WHAT WILL YOU DO AND
HOW WILL YOU DO IT?

Good project planning pays off. It is the method by which the team figures out how to make the project happen. It makes a project team more effective in achieving its aims and more capable of acquiring and using the right resources and methods. Good planning means selecting achievable aims, designing feasible means, managing the workload, making the best use of everyone's talents and establishing the basis for good decision making.

In this chapter we focus on the process of planning what needs to be done to achieve the project goals, and how it will be done. We bring together project planning methods with service planning methods developed in the health and community services sector, and give a step-by-step outline for writing a good project plan and the issues that need to be resolved at this stage.

WHY PLAN AT ALL?

Planning is working out what to do before action is taken (Rubin and Rubin 1992:389); every project management writer stresses that good project design and planning are critical to project success. The project plan is a blueprint for the entire project, and is the guide for future project activities.

Usually, however, there is pressure to get a project done quickly, and it can be very tempting to get on with the actual work of the project as soon as possible and either avoid planning or pay it lip service only.

There are many reasons for resistance to planning, and they include:

- Planning can be difficult (it forces people to think, it requires negotiation, collaboration and decision making).
- Many people believe that plans are a waste of time because inevitably plans change during the course of a project.
- For most people planning is not as satisfying as actually doing the work and getting quick results.
- People lack the skills for planning.
- A project plan can be seen as an organisational straightjacket rather than a working tool (adapted from Maylor 1996:46).

Every person we interviewed emphasised the importance of good planning. There are some very powerful reasons for taking up this challenge. Failure to start with a clear plan almost guarantees that your project will not be successful because there is not enough definition of what you are going to do or how you are going to do it. Without a project plan (addressing 'what, who, how, when and at what cost'), and without this plan being agreed to or signed off, it is likely that there will be general confusion, lack of common understanding, higher costs, and a lot of stress and discontent (Webster 1999:14–15). Of course, the size and nature of the project determine how elaborate the plan needs to be, and how much time and energy are needed to prepare it.

It needs to be recognised that the time taken for planning and development can be anywhere up to a third of the total project timeframe and can equal the time spent on project implementation.

PROCESSES AND ACTIVITIES OF PLANNING: THE RATIONAL APPROACH

Because project planning is so critical in mainstream project management theory, there are many different terms in use and several models. However, all these models, in common with service planning in the health and community services sector, are based on the rational planning framework. That is, planning proceeds in a logical order through the elements of the plan, described in service planning language as rationale, goals, objectives, strategies, timelines, resources and evaluation. The steps and terms used in the mainstream project management literature are a little different, and the jargon can be confusing, but the logic will be familiar. Table 1 outlines the processes involved.

Before we work through the steps and methods of planning, we need to recognise that for many newcomers to planning it is precisely the rational basis behind it that makes them sceptical. Working life is hardly ever as logical as the plan, and people act in ways which are not imagined in rationales, goals and strategies. They may even set out to deliberately undermine or sabotage projects.

Sometimes circumstances mean that a project cannot 'start at the beginning', or that the rationale for the project has to be assembled after other decisions have already been made, or that the timeline is patently not achievable. Sometimes circumstances change during the life of the project. Sometimes the project team makes promises to stakeholders which it cannot keep, or the executive has another good idea which changes the project scope.

The value of planning can seem doubtful for soft projects (defined as complex tasks aimed at intangible results). Most organisational change and service development projects have at least some of the characteristics of soft projects. That is, compared to building projects, for example, the objectives and scope are more likely to change after commencement, costs are more difficult to estimate, and the logical relationships between activities are not as concrete (McElroy 1996:327). However, experience with such projects (arguably the majority in the health and community services sector) indicates that planning is especially valuable in conditions of uncertainty.

It is also important to remember that planning is often an iterative process. For example, the project may start with a clear plan, but the objectives might change when strategies are better developed in the early stages of implementation. New possibilities might open up, or anticipated resources might shrink. There can be frequent movement between planning and implementing activities, particularly at the beginning of a project.

Projects in all fields experience unforeseen problems that require change to the plan, some of them similar to those outlined above. For example, engineers need to be concerned about things like rocks or tunnels under the ground right where the bridge pylons need to go, and they use contingency planning in response (see the section on risk management later in this chapter).

Table 1: Project planning process and activities

Components of the project plan	Activities
Project charter	Defining the goals, objectives and strategies
Scope planning and definition	Defining how big the project is going to be, what is within or outside the boundaries of the project Identifying stakeholders Sometimes called a Statement of Work (SOW)
Project structures	Locating the project in the organisation structure Designing project committees and decision making Involving consumers
Activity definition, sequencing and timing	Development of the Work Breakdown Structure (WBS), i.e. the project tasks and activities, and the relationships between the activities Estimation of how long each task will take
Schedule development	Plotting project tasks against a timeline including project phases and decision points, deadlines, milestones and critical pathways
Human resource planning	Role of project manager Identifying the human resources required for the project Building the project team
Resources, cost estimating and budgeting	Defining and estimating the cost of the resources required for the project, and development of the project budget
Risk management planning	Identifying what could go wrong (the risks), and assessing how likely it is that things go wrong Planning for contingencies and a process for resolving them
Project quality plan	Defining the quality standards to be met by the project outcomes Systems for monitoring quality
Organisational planning	Project logistics Project communication plan for informing stakeholders, reporting progress Project information systems

Source: Adapted from PMBOK (PMI 2000:3334)

The key point is that hardly anything goes exactly according to plan, but having a plan helps you to deal with the chaos of real life and still get there in the end. Not having a plan is like negotiating the freeways of an unknown city without a map. You might be able to see the landmark you are headed for, but you are likely to end up somewhere completely different if you don't know the route.

FOUNDATION OF THE PROJECT PLAN: THE PROJECT CHARTER

The project charter (or 'project scope', 'definition', 'statement of work') is the first key element of the plan. Essentially, the charter could be described as the 'rules of the game' (Verzuh 1999:55) by which the project runs. Everything else in the plan is based on achieving the project as defined in the project charter. Getting the charter right is a critical first step in planning, and this is where the creative thinking is concentrated and the project design is fundamentally set. When projects are undertaken by external consultants, the project charter will be a key part of the contract.

In Chapter 4 we addressed the setting of clear goals and the writing of a project proposal, noting that these steps are often necessary for project funding applications or internal approvals which enable the proponents to proceed with further development. The proposal is essentially a rough outline of the project plan which establishes the overall purpose or goals of the project and other key characteristics. The project charter is an expansion of the front end of the proposal, and the key steps are confirming the goals, developing objectives, outlining strategies, defining the scope (that is, the limits), defining deliverables and identifying key stakeholders.

In this section, we work through the steps involved in completing the project charter. We have amalgamated two of the project stories we collected as part of our research, and constructed a single story to illustrate the key steps. (Please note that MET teams, the subject of the story, are real, but this story is not the real story of their beginning.) The starting point is a common one: someone with a good idea for solving a difficult but worthwhile problem.

Developing a MET team: the goal

The head of the intensive care unit of a large suburban hospital was convinced that he had a good idea to

---

improve outcomes for the hospital's patients. The idea, which had been initiated in another hospital, is known as a medical emergency team. The purpose is to change the way hospital staff respond to instability in patients' vital signs (respiration rate, heart rate and others), changes which indicate that they are getting dangerously sick. The traditional procedure is that the ward nurse alerts the resident medical officer, who assesses the patient and if appropriate alerts the registrar, who in turn responds and may need to contact the consultant or senior doctor. These steps are designed to ensure that the senior treating doctor makes important decisions about patient care, a good principle designed to protect the quality of care as well as enable learning by junior doctors, and one which is still effective for many purposes. But the system was designed in another era, when hospitals did not have intensive care units.

The intended change essentially circumvents the normal protocol for responding to instability in key observations by empowering ward nurses to call the MET team—a doctor and nurse from ICU—instead of going up through the medical chain of command. The ICU director decided to initiate a project which would trial the MET team idea and methodically evaluate the results. His goal was clear:

To trial a medical emergency team in this hospital and test its effectiveness.

Operationalising the goal: objectives

Once the aim or goal is clear (there may be more than one but, ideally, each project should be able to be expressed as a single, concrete goal), it may be a good idea to break it down into objectives. Objectives are more concrete expressions of the aim, and are desired endpoints or outcomes in themselves. Whether this step is needed will depend on the size and complexity of the project—sometimes the aim is so straightforward that it does not need to be broken down into objectives. Objectives can be seen as steps along the way to achieving the goal; they should clarify rather than broaden the goal and, like the goal, need to be achievable and measurable.

The MET team: objectives

The next steps for the director of ICU were to get support from the hospital's general manager, and find the resources needed to implement the project. He also knew that there would be some opposition, and concerns about things like nurses taking more responsibility and relationships between the ICU doctors and others.

The general manager was supportive—she was keen for the hospital to develop a reputation for research in improving health care delivery, and to boost its effectiveness through quality improvement. There was an upcoming round of grants for quality improvement projects, and the director decided to develop the idea as a submission for funding, with the general manager's help. This meant the preparation of a project proposal, so a workshop was held with a small number of allies— a physician, the nursing head of ICU and the hospital's director of nursing, as well as the quality manager. The group was very interested in the idea, and also sceptical about its feasibility, but decided it was worth a try. Their first task was to confirm the goal and develop objectives. After much discussion they expanded the goal, and after gathering more information and contacting the overseas hospital they developed objectives:

Goal: To trial a medical emergency team in this hospital and test its effectiveness in reducing mortality and critical events.

Objectives:
1. To determine the parameters of instability in vital signs which are good indicators of risk of critical events (defined as in-hospital cardiac arrest and unplanned admission to ICU) and death.
2. To develop and test a protocol, based on the defined parameters, for calling a MET team; and for the management of continuing care and communication with all treating doctors.
3. To identify and train MET personnel, and establish the team.

> 4. To design and test a training program for ward nursing staff.
> 5. To evaluate the cost and effectiveness of the MET concept, using comprehensive baseline and trial data on the incidence of critical events, and the associated morbidity and mortality, complemented by financial analysis of costs and savings.

There would have been many tasks underlying these objectives—for example, 'to arrange a meeting with the senior medical staff to inform them of this project proposal and seek their support'—but this is a means rather than a result and belongs in the work program, not among the objectives. Developing the five objectives was a challenge in itself, and required some hard thinking about the elements of the problem and how it was likely to be solved. The team needed to investigate feasibility (such questions as, 'Could the ICU cope with admissions arising from MET calls?') and agree on the definition of a critical event. They also needed to consider the perspectives of stakeholders, be sensitive to the requirements of the funding agency, and think creatively in order to deal with all these considerations in this first phase of project design.

In developing objectives there are three useful things to remember:

- Language—use action verbs; for example, 'improving', 'providing', 'developing'.
- Focus each objective on one specific outcome or deliverable.
- Make statements of objectives realistic, that is, measurable and achievable (Brody 2000:63).

The difference between an aim and an objective (or a strategy and a task) may be largely a function of where you are sitting. For the CEO of a large community agency, winning a particular government contract may be an objective, but for the staff whose service or jobs depend on that contract it will be seen as the primary aim.

Strategies: how the objectives will be achieved

The simplest way to think about the strategies for a project is to consider each objective (or sometimes the aim) and ask how will it be achieved? What needs to be done?

The MET project: strategies

As awareness of the proposal spread in the hospital, debate about the wisdom of setting up a MET team, and about the real impact on patients, also grew. Some interesting problems were raised, like the need to ensure respect for the wishes of patients who had given instructions that they were not to be resuscitated should they get into trouble. How should these instructions be interpreted under a MET protocol? The proponents were alert to the need to listen carefully and consider the implications of all concerns. They had two goals for this process—to use the debate to improve the design, and to reassure the stakeholders that their interests would be looked after and they would be able to have their say throughout the trial.

The funding submission guidelines required that the proposal outline how the project would achieve its objectives, so the next step was to write the strategies. The director drafted strategies for each of the objectives—the key strategies relating to the first two are shown here:

1   To determine the parameters of instability in vital signs which are good indicators of risk of critical events (defined as in-hospital cardiac arrest and unplanned admission to ICU).
1.1 Starting with the parameters used by the overseas hospital, collect data on the readings for all patients who experienced a critical event in the last year (using medical records).
1.2 Use this data and other research to identify whether the signs, and the critical levels of instability in each, are robust and reliable enough for use in this hospital.
2   To develop and test a protocol, based on the defined parameters, for calling a MET team and for the management of continuing care and communication with all treating doctors.
2.1 Draft a protocol, in collaboration with senior clinical nurses, ICU staff and consultant doctors.
2.2 Circulate the protocol to senior nursing and medical forums for comment and analyse the comments for both technical and work practice concerns.

103

2.3 Send the protocol to three identified experts (two internal medicine and one intensive care) for review.

2.4 Draft and circulate a proposal for a steering committee and consultation mechanisms, and analyse feedback to identify the key representatives of stakeholder groups (both supportive and opposed) and their key concerns.

2.5 Establish a steering committee early in the project to ensure that stakeholder issues can be managed. Appoint a senior clinician to chair the committee.

The project plan should describe the strategies in enough detail for the project team, stakeholders and decision makers to understand how the project will achieve its goals and objectives. Not every project needs all three levels of goals, objectives and strategies. However, note that among these three levels, it is the objectives that can be skipped, never the goals or the strategies.

Drawing a line around it: project scope

How big is this project going to be? What activities are going to be included or excluded? How does the project fit with the operational activities of the organisation? These are essentially questions regarding project scope, and they have a huge bearing on the size and potentially the success of the project. If a project scope is not clearly defined in the planning stage it can quickly get out of control. According to the Standish Group (Hayes 2002), only one in five of all major projects actually meets schedule or budgetary goals. Many of the reasons that the money and time objectives of a project are not met relate to how the project was designed and how the boundaries around it were drawn.

The MET project: scope

In this project the borders were pretty clearly defined. The patients in the hospital were the target group, and the parameters for calling the team established the limits on who would receive MET care. The following scope limits were defined:

- The trial will operate for a period of one year.
- The protocol will not be changed during that time, unless ethical issues emerge.
- The trial will not be expanded to other hospitals in the larger health service.

Defining deliverables

Consulting contracts often include a detailed statement of the products or outputs of the contract that will be handed over or otherwise given to the client at the end of the contract. The deliverables are simply the answer to the question 'What will this project deliver?' and they might include a report, a piece of software, a training package or any product commissioned as part of the project. This concept can also be useful for internal projects in forcing a clear delineation of the product or output in even more concrete terms than the goals or objectives.

The MET team: deliverables

The concept of deliverables was a new one for the hospital team, but the submission guidelines asked 'What practical products or services will the project hand over to the sponsoring organisation at the completion of the funding period?'

The deliverables were defined in answer to this question as:

- An agreed and tested protocol for responding to critical events in patients at this hospital.
- A training manual for clinical ward nursing staff in safe use of the protocol.
- A procedure manual for MET team members.
- An evaluation of the effectiveness of the MET team, based on comprehensive data about patient outcomes, including and economic evaluation.
- A costing for the outgoing operation of the MET team, and an analysis of the net cost and benefit to the hospital.

Identifying stakeholders

Stakeholders are the individuals and organisations which are actively involved in the project, or whose interests may be affected as a result of the project, or who may exert influence over the project and its results (PMI 2000:16). In the planning phase, the project team needs to identify the stakeholders, plan for their engagement and identify the interests and allegiances that can affect the project. While this is not always easy to do, projects will have stakeholders that fall into the following categories:

■ Sponsor or champion—person or group that provides the finances and executive management support for the project.

■ Project manager—the person nominated to manage the project.

■ Customers or users—the person, group or organisation that consumes or uses the project's product or outcomes.

■ Partners and allies—the external organisations and individuals whose contribution or support is needed, or whose opposition needs to be managed.

■ Performing organisation or department—the organisation or department whose employees are most directly involved in doing the work.

■ Project team members—the group performing the work of the project.

Once stakeholders are identified, it is useful to consider the impact that a particular stakeholder group may have on the project, and how they will be managed. Stakeholders may have the power to veto or approve, delay, facilitate, derail or guide a project.

The MET project: stakeholder analysis

It was clear to everyone from the beginning that there were powerful stakeholders who could exert great influence on the MET project's chances of success. Significant support and cooperation would be needed, and there were many old friends and enemies, allies, competitors and idealists who would all need to be managed. A high-level stakeholder analysis was done of several vitally important players who could easily go either way. The initial list (and the confidential analysis) included:

- *Medical staff:* Likely to see the change as a criticism of their previous practice; important for them to have ownership of the project and get credit for improved outcomes. New professor of medicine a likely ally, because of research aspect and her clinical interests.
- *Nursing staff:* Being asked to take on additional responsibility, and risk disapproval of medical colleagues; will need to feel safe and supported, and to maintain control over their own practice; need to keep union representatives informed.
- *Health Department:* Likely to support the project because of clinical value and rigour of evaluation strategy; important to recognise their contributions.
- *Intensive Care Faculty of College of Physicians:* Likely to support, but probably best not to involve them because might raise the hackles of other medical staff.

A simple 2 × 2 map of the stakeholders is a useful planning tool which can help with preparation for active management of stakeholder issues in the implementation phase, as represented in Figure 4.

Figure 4: Stakeholder mapping

	Not important	Very important
Hinder	Problematic — need to be monitored	Antagonistic — need active strategies for management
Support	Low priority — keep on side	Champions — work with them

To complete the mapping exercise, stakeholders are identified and categorised as to whether they are supportive or opposed to the project, and rated for their relative importance—that is, the amount of power or influence they can exert on the project. Strategies for managing the way the stakeholders engage with the project can then be developed, with the aim of minimising opposition and maximising support. Stakeholder management is a vital issue, and we return to it later in this chapter (see the section on project committees).

WHEN ENOUGH PLANNING IS ENOUGH

With the goals, objectives, strategies, scope and key stakeholders defined, the project charter is now complete. In the rest of the project plan, all the major resources and methods required to give life to the project charter are worked out and documented. The length and complexity of the plan is primarily dependent on the size and scope of the project. Some organisations have templates or defined processes for the development of the project plan, and may stipulate what should be included in the document. Completed project plans can vary from about five pages to about 50 (or even larger for large and complex projects).

The more carefully thought out the plan, the more likely it is that the project will stay on track and the fewer surprises (or crises) there will be in the implementation and closing/evaluation phases. The energy spent in developing the plan to a sufficient level of detail, in collaboration with stakeholders, will result in greater understanding by all of what is expected of them as part of the project, and thus avoid, or at least identify and make more manageable, a lot of potential conflict. But it is also possible to do too much planning, and get too worried about details.

Maylor (1996:46–7) warns of the dangers of planning for planning's sake, and points out that a well-balanced plan will guide the actions of the project team without the need to define to the last detail what each person is doing every minute of the day.

Case 10: 'Detailitis'

The concept was quite attractive—the establishment of a health check clinic that would meet the needs of business and industry executives, and serve as a feeder for the hospital's cardiac program. So far so good. This was, however, where the rough planning stopped and the group succumbed to the virus that plagues so many projects at this point—detailitis. The discussions were waylaid by the need to have the width of the clinic doors trolley-compatible, the colour of the décor and the pricing structure of visits to the clinic. No matter that three other similar clinics had been set up in the inner metropolitan area and were competing heavily for business (adapted from Maylor 1996:48).

PROJECT STRUCTURE: PLANNING FOR EFFECTIVE OPERATIONS

With the project charter developed and agreed, there are five strands of planning which can commence simultaneously—planning the project structures, planning the activities and resources, planning to manage risk and quality, planning project logistics and planning for evaluation. If the project is a small one, some of these headings might need only half a page in the project plan, but even small projects benefit from appropriate attention to each component.

This section focuses on the placement of the project in the organisation, and the methods of engaging stakeholders and maximising support.

Locating the project in the organisational structure

Planning for the location of the project within the organisational structure, and specifying its reporting lines and access to decision makers, can prevent unhelpful project politics later on. The project manager's role will likewise be made easier if their place in the structure and the decision-making systems is clear and appropriate to the task.

There are a number of ways in which projects can be structured within organisations. There is no one right answer, it is rather a question of finding the best balance of advantages and disadvantages. Functional structures (where the project is 'owned' by the unit or department most involved, the normal employer of most of the project team) have several advantages. They tend to have maximum flexibility in the use of their staff; individual experts can be utilised for many different projects; and specialists can be grouped to share knowledge and experience. The functional structure also provides a career path for individuals—doing well in the project can help them advance in the hierarchy (Meredith and Mantel 2000).

However, a number of problems can also arise in this kind of structure. The project may suffer from a lack of focus and attention when it is competing with ongoing tasks, and the management of the unit may not be well placed to cope with project characteristics such as more urgent timelines. The project may require the unit to work with other parts of the organisation or another service provider in a way which is at odds with its ongoing relationships, or staff not engaged in the project may feel exploited (Lientz and Rea 1998).

When projects within a functional structure come unstuck, the typical outcome is that they slip down the priority list and are delayed, downgraded or allowed to fade away. The best predictors of success in this structure are that the project is championed by the unit manager, the team has authority to make decisions about the project, and the project deals with an issue which matters to the staff in their daily work.

The main alternative structure is the matrix system, where project staff are drawn from functional units, thus cutting across the organisation structure for the life of the project. The project manager reports to a senior manager in the role of project sponsor, and the team members report to the project manager at least for the purposes of the project. The advantages of a matrix structure are that projects and project teams are given a strong identity within the organisation and resources are allocated accordingly. The downsides can include conflicts between line managers and project staff, undermining of the traditional organisation and unclear roles and responsibilities (Alsene 1998). Case 11 illustrates the problem.

Case 11: Conflict between projects and operations

A women's health service had grown and developed through successful tendering for a number of projects and attracting new project funds on the basis of its successful track record.

A matrix structure had emerged by default rather than planning. The project management staff had their own ways of doing things; this frustrated the core staff, who felt that the project staff were receiving special treatment and did not work within the guiding values of the women's health service. This was made worse by the fact that the project staff were often based in large partner organisations and tended to identify strongly with these partners.

The situation came to a head when the organisation held a strategic planning workshop for all staff. It became clear that the staff were becoming factionalised in two groups, the 'old core staff', committed to the ideals and philosophies of the centre, and the 'new project staff', who were committed to their projects but had little commitment to the parent organisation. Management was forced to put strategic planning on hold while it dealt with the structural and cultural issues.

Designing project committees and decision-making structures

Steering committees, advisory committees and reference groups can help to make or break projects. A steering committee usually implies some level of control and ownership over the project, and literally steers the project in the direction it wishes it to go. Reference groups and advisory committees usually imply a less hands-on relationship, seeing themselves as providing advice and support and helping the project to work well. The design of project committees, and their ways of working, will depend partly on whether the project is internally focused (for example, the reorganisation of care processes) or externally focused (for example, the development of an area health plan).

Chapman and Davey (1997) identify a number of critical issues in establishing the project management structure for an externally-focused health planning project:

- clarifying the role and decision-making capacities of the project committee;
- gaining appropriate representation on the committee (recruiting suitably influential members who are comfortable with the participatory processes);
- identifying an effective chairperson who can facilitate interactive meetings;
- motivating members to persist with an often complex and demanding process;
- ensuring community participation if relevant; and
- securing participation by other parts of the organisation (1997:87).

Our respondents also spoke about the difficulties of committees being dominated by particular personalities or people who had 'their own barrows to push', and the way such individuals could derail projects. In the Queensland health planning experience there were a number of factors that enhanced the way the committees worked. These were:

- personal contact by the project team between meetings;
- interactive meeting procedures that allowed shared ownership of the project;
- the flexibility to change direction if necessary;
- regular and timely correspondence between meetings;
- time for social networking within the scheduled meetings and a focus on hospitality;
- public recognition of the work done by the committee (within and external to the organisation);
- coordination of strategy development by committee members; and
- the development of a sense of congruence between the goals of the plan and the professional needs and expectations of the committee members (1997:87).

The PRINCE method deals more extensively with the issue of project direction by a steering committee or board than many of the mainstream project models (perhaps reflecting the origins of this model in the public sector), in ways that seem useful for internal projects. Stakeholder management in internal projects has its own challenges—for example, there is often no defined 'client' to accept or reject outcomes. Individuals may have roles in both supplying inputs to the project and using its outputs, and the interests of the stakeholders are sometimes seen as a kind of zero sum game—that is, one person's win is another's loss. In these circumstances, stakeholder paralysis is a real threat to projects which seek to change the way business is done.

In the PRINCE approach an empowered steering committee is chaired by the project sponsor (or the executive in charge of the project). It takes responsibility for signing off the various stages of the project and for its final outcome. It makes decisions that are needed at this level along the way, and acts as a sounding board for the project manager and the team.

The committee is made up of senior representatives of the major stakeholder groups; that is, those who will use or work with the results of the project, and those who are required to deliver services or capacity to support the project outcomes. A deliberate distinction is made between 'suppliers' and 'users': the suppliers are asked to monitor cost and feasibility, while the users are asked to focus on functionality and quality. For example, in a project which aims to introduce a new patient administration system into an emergency department, the computing services department of the hospital has a strong interest, along with the emergency clinicians (medical and nursing), the medical records staff and the clerical staff of the department. The IT department and the administrative staff would be asked to take the role of suppliers on the committee, and their vested interest in having a system which is efficient, easy to maintain and to service is recognised. The clinicians are asked to take the role of user, and their interest in ease of use and quality of data is recognised. The health information (medical records) staff might need to have a seat at both ends of this table.

We suggest that the terms of reference of the committee are considered at the planning stage, and that time is taken (perhaps in the early stages of implementation) to develop and finalise them properly. Any potentially difficult issues should be dealt with up front in a business-like way to prevent them becoming really difficult and heated issues further down the track.

Involving consumers

Consumer representation on the steering committee, or other project consultative bodies, can add value in several ways. The following factors are relevant to this decision:

- Will the project have a direct impact on care for patients and clients?
- Is the relevant service one which has ongoing relationships with its consumers?
- Will the rights of consumers (for example, to privacy, or self-determination) be affected by the project?
- Are there issues of equity of access and appropriateness of service for population groups with special needs (for example, disabilities or mental illness, or for indigenous people)?
- Are there established advocacy or interest groups who can offer expertise and who might affect (positively or negatively) the success of the project?

If the answer to any of these questions is 'yes', we would suggest that the real question is 'Is there any justification for not involving consumers?' The next question is to determine how consumers can be involved. If the project has a steering committee on which stakeholders are represented, then that is probably the place. But it may be that there are other more effective methods of engagement, depending on the project.

For further consideration of these issues, there is a good guide (called 'Improving health services through consumer participation: A resource guide for organisations') available at the website *http://www.participateinhealth.org.au/clearinghouse/* (Commonwealth of Australia 2000).

PLANNING PROJECT ACTIVITIES AND RESOURCES

The next area of planning gets to the core of the work program, and planning for the resources that will be needed to achieve it. This section addresses planning tasks and activities, scheduling them, staging the project if necessary, planning the team and other resources that will be needed, and their costs. The range of tools and methods discussed below (including scheduling, work breakdown structures and charting) enable the project manager and the team to:

- Document all the tasks and activities that have to be completed.
- See an overview of the project tasks against a timeline.
- Identify the resources required to complete the tasks.

- See the relationships and dependencies between the tasks.
- Identify milestones within the project (a milestone is a significant event or major point of progress in the course of a project).
- Identify how long the project will take and any deadlines (or critical points) within the project.
- Manage change and delay in the completion of project tasks.

Project tasks and activities: what needs to be done?

'A journey of a thousand miles starts from beneath one's feet.' (*Lao Tse 1963:125*)

Project strategies cannot work unless there is a clear action plan, with the necessary staff, resources and equipment at hand. It is sometimes useful to pretest strategies, perhaps through a pilot. For example, if you are constructing a questionnaire to use with a particular group, it could be pretested on a similar group, to discover whether the questions make sense, flow in a logical order and extract the kind of information you are hoping to find. If you are intending to carry out a project that involves a group of medical specialists, it is often useful to speak to a couple of representatives first to explore the ways that the group might think about an issue, so as to be informed about likely attitudes and issues. These activities should be identified in the planning stages and written into the plan.

The activities and tasks of a project need to be defined and broken down into manageable chunks. The simplest way to do this is to start with the aims, strategies and deliverables identified in the project charter, break them up using subheadings and expand on them in a list format. In project management terms this is called creating a work breakdown structure (WBS). In developing the WBS it can be difficult to think of all the tasks that need to be done, and the ideas will probably flow faster if it is done by the team or a working group rather than an individual.

There are many techniques and rules of thumb for developing the WBS which can help with sizing the tasks, defining the relationships between them and other technical aspects. Some of the texts listed in Chapter 3 describe this process in detail.

Scheduling and scheduling tools

Next, task subheadings are sorted into a logical sequence, in other words, what needs to happen first, second, third, and so on, and the time needed for each task is estimated (or often 'guesstimated'). Estimating how long each task will take and plotting the tasks against a timeline is called scheduling.

Figure 5 is an example in chart form of the activities and timing that might be used in the development and conduct of a community survey.

Figure 5: A simple work breakdown structure (WBS)

Activity	Timing
Project start date	Day 1
1. Carry out literature review	Day 2 to 20
2. Arrange visits for piloting	Day 15 to 20
3. Prepare questionnaire	Day 21 to 30
4. Pilot questionnaire	Day 33 to 40
5. Review questionnaire	Day 33 to 45
6. Deliver questionnaire	Day 46 to 60
7. Analyse results	Day 65 to 80
8. Write report	Day 2 to 87
9. Presentation of report	Day 90

The same information is often shown in graphical form in a Gantt chart, which plots the activities (in rows) against the timeline (in columns), thus showing the relationships between them. Gantt charts can also show the resources required for a particular task or activity, the relationships between tasks, milestones and baselines, and can be used to track planned and actual progress (Meredith and Mantel 2000). Figure 6 presents the information in Figure 5 as a Gantt chart.

The Gantt chart is one of the most commonly used methods of presenting schedule information (and of charting actual progress) and is synonymous with project management. For a simple project a Gantt chart may be hand drawn (or charted on a whiteboard); for more complex projects it may be developed on a computer (using,

Figure 6: A simple Gantt chart

	Task Name	Duration	April 2003	May 2003	June 2003	July 2003
1	**Literature review**	20 days				
2	⊟ **Conduct survey**	39 days				
3	Prepare questionnaire	10 days				
4	Pilot questionnaire	7 days				
5	Review questionnaire	7 days				
6	Interviews	15 days				
7	**Analyse results**	15 days				
8	⊟ **Write report**	65 days				
9	Structure & outline	5 days				
10	First draft	27 days				
11	Second draft	12 days				18/07
12	**Presentation of report**	0 days				

for example, Microsoft Project software). Gantt charts are a very useful tool in both the planning and implementation phases of the project because they are simple, easily understood and very effective for showing the status of a task or group of tasks against the schedule. Their limitations include that they can be difficult to update if there are lots of changes and they can become unmanageable in more complex projects.

The many other project management charting and scheduling techniques include network diagrams, critical path analysis (which shows the critical tasks and times for the project to meet a deadline), and the program evaluation and review technique (PERT—one of the first formal methods developed for scheduling projects). They are not often used in health and community services, other than in some building and IT projects, because there is not the same focus on managing technical tasks and resources concurrently. Descriptions and tips on how to use them are included in many texts.

Planning decision points and project stages

Innovation projects, aimed at achieving change in the way care is delivered to patients/clients or the way that business processes work, are often better handled in stages. This is helpful when there are major unknowns which can only be answered as the project progresses. Designing projects in stages, where redesign

117

in the light of learnings from the previous stage is a planned strategy, can be an essential aid to maintaining both momentum and control.

Some of the breaks between stages may be designated 'go/no go' points, where the answers to important questions can mean that the project should be abandoned. At other times the answers will bring the need for significant choices among alternatives.

Staging of this kind can also assist in creating a more comfortable framework for the consideration of major changes. The establishment of planned times and methods for deciding whether particular designs work, and whether the benefits and costs are in the right balance, can make it easier for people to agree to proceed with projects about which they have misgivings. For example, it may be much more acceptable to the staff of a pathology service to move high-volume tests to a centralised core laboratory (and out of specialised laboratories) if they know that there will be detailed modelling and testing of the proposed solutions, including rosters and staffing levels, before implementation begins.

In order to design a project in stages, the key decision points need to be identified very early in planning, along with the decision makers, and the information they will use. Important meetings may need to be timed accordingly (while allowing for some slippage). In effect, each stage needs its own plan. While this may sound daunting, it can in fact make the task easier because the planning is broken into manageable pieces, and it allows more flexibility in the planning for later stages.

We come back to the question of how decisions external to the team are to be made in the sections on reporting structures and committees below.

Planning for human resource needs

'People make projects happen.' (*Verzuh 1999*)

Working out the human resource requirements and how to build the project team are critical tasks for most projects, and some steps can be taken at the planning stage. The project charter and the detailed list of tasks and timings are the starting point.

Often writing the detailed project plan is the first task of the newly appointed project manager, so some of the key questions below may have already been answered:

- What kind of skills are needed to achieve this project?
- Which of those skills are needed by the manager?
- What other people with particular skills are needed, and how much of their time, or how many of them?
- How will technical expertise not available among team members be brought in?
- What process will be used for selecting the project manager and other team members?
- How much authority over team members will the manager have?

This is the stage when organisations that have nurtured project capability and skills within the organisation will be seeing the benefits of their investment. On the other hand, contracting for project management and team members may be a necessary, or desirable, strategy.

The role of project sponsor

The sponsor or champion is somebody senior in the organisation who authorises the project and usually fulfils most or all of these functions:

- Chairing the project steering committee or working group.
- Acting as the supervisor of the project manager.
- Ensuring that the project team has good access to people and resources across the organisation, as needed by the project.
- Signing off (sometimes on behalf of the committee) on major decisions or variations as part of the project, and receiving the final report.

If the project is contracted out, the equivalent role is generally played by the person who is 'the client' (who may be the person who signs the contract), and the functions are similar. The sponsor may have been identified in the early stages of the project, and then the remaining tasks are to define the role and document it as part of the plan.

Working with consultants

Because of the individual uniqueness of projects it is rare for an organisation to have all the necessary skills in-house for a major project (Healy 1997:15). This is as true of human services as any other area, so that consultants and temporary specialist staff are often engaged either to work directly on a project or to back-fill operational positions. The nature of the relationship between contracted staff and the project manager or sponsor needs to be well planned and communicated.

Consultants can add real value to a project by bringing high-order skills, up-to-date knowledge from elsewhere in your field, the objectivity of the outsider and a greater freedom to deliver uncomfortable messages or challenge the prevailing culture. On the negative side, working with consultants can be a knowledge drain for the organisation. To prevent this the contract can include a requirement for the consultants to transfer knowledge and skills, and to hand over all the 'intelligence' gathered as part of the project (in the form of briefings as well as organised files). This can ensure that the organisation gets value for money from the consultancy, and also reduces the likelihood of future dependency on a particular consultant or firm.

Resources, cost estimating and budgeting

In this part of the plan resources required for the project are identified, their costs estimated and the project budget developed. Estimating is forecasting the future, trying to predict the time and money necessary to produce a result (Verzuh 1999:153). Volumes of information have been written about the intricacies of estimating project costs and time, together with numerous techniques, computer and mathematical models (apportioning, parametric estimates, etc.). Verzuh (1999:153–87) gives a good overview of these techniques.

Essentially, the following resources in the project must be planned for, and their costs estimated:

- The staff (labour) required to do the work of the project, both within and outside the organisation. The time of the project manager and all project team members, even if they are salaried staff, should be included, along with any additional expertise that may have to be 'purchased' in the form of legal advice, consultants, statisticians, technical writers, and so on.
- Equipment, services and materials required for the project; that is, the direct costs of setting up the project office, and all consumables required to deliver the outcomes of the project. Once again, it is sometimes difficult for one person to come

up with a comprehensive list, and team brainstorming is often the fastest way to develop a list and then to estimate the cost of each item.

There are a number of pitfalls in the estimating process. Because estimates are often based not on information but on best guesses, people tend to under- or overestimate. It may not be necessary to get an actual quotation for every single item, but your guesses should be informed. When asked to guess how much or how long, enthusiasts and supporters may minimise the effort or resources required. Someone disinclined toward or not supportive of a project (or just very averse to risk) will tend to overestimate the time or cost and perhaps jeopardise the project's very existence.

The question of how many of the costs to include also arises, and the answer depends on things such as how the project will be funded and the organisation's approach to cost accounting. Costing may be marginal, that is, only including the extra costs directly incurred because the project is happening. Another way of thinking about marginal costs is in the negative—cost only the resources that would not be used if the project wasn't happening. Alternatively, full costing would include all the direct costs of the project (that is, costs of all resources used by the project, including, for example, light, power and cleaning, all staff time attributable to the project) plus an allowance for overheads (the CEO's salary, the payroll system, etc.).

The initial estimate may have been prepared as part of a funding application, or for the first stage of project approval. In any case, more accurate estimating is part of the process of developing a detailed budget, which should be part of the project plan.

Developing the project budget

Once a project is approved, a budget that details all proposed items of expenditure (including salaries) is required. In the implementation phase the budget becomes the primary document for controlling costs. As far as possible, costs should be based not on guesstimates but on data gathered from the organisation's finance and payroll systems, together with quotations for any externally provided products or services.

The budget format depends largely on the project itself and on the norm for the organisation, but a simple spreadsheet can be used to list all project expenditure items. Expenditure items may be grouped according to labour (staff) or non-labour (equipment/ materials) items, fixed versus variable expenses, internal versus external or initial versus ongoing costs.

PLANNING FOR RISK AND QUALITY

The project plan should include sections dealing with risk (What might go wrong? How will it be handled?) and quality (What are the standards the project outcomes must meet?). Decisions made in this stage of the planning might affect other aspects of the plan. Checking these interactions is part of the planning process.

Risk management and contingency planning

'All project management is risk management.' (*Verzuh 1999*)

In undertaking any project there is a risk that something will happen to jeopardise either the budget, the quality, the timelines, the stakeholder support or the achievement of the project's aims and its sustainability. Good planning includes a process for identifying the risks associated with the project, under-standing the severity of the risk and planning contingencies.

Risk management is the means by which uncertainty is systematically managed to increase the likelihood of meeting project objectives (Verzuh 1999:79). The aim of risk management is to control and reduce risk. The first step in the process is to analyse the project to identify sources of risk. This is perhaps best achieved by consultation or a meeting with key stakeholders to ask the critical questions and then create a risk management plan. What can happen to cause problems for this project? Will there be enough staff to cover the roster? Will the new radio-therapy machine be delivered on time? Will industrial activity impact on the timeline? Will there be a change of government policy or corporate leadership?

After defining the possible risks, including their potential negative impact on the project (that is, what is the result if the risk happens?), each risk can be assigned a probability rating. Then a strategy (also called a contingency) can be developed to respond to the risks and reduce possible damage to the project and the organisation. To manage project risk effectively, a risk management plan (sometimes called a log or a matrix) should be developed as part of the planning process.

Figure 7: A risk management plan example

Risk and potential impact	Risk level	Design features to reduce likelihood of occurrence	Contingencies to reduce impact (if it occurs)	Responsibility
Community not willing to complete questionnaire	Medium	Involve staff that are familiar to community	Survey additional community representatives	Project officer

Source: Logframe matrix model

Project risks are classified according to the likelihood of their occurring and the seriousness of the consequences if they do occur. The likelihood may range from rare (for example, the chances of an earthquake) to almost certain (for example, the chances of minor vandalism in a carpark) whereas the consequences may range from insignificant to catastrophic. The risk level is assigned by plotting the item against these two attributes of risk in a risk matrix (see Figure 8).

Figure 8: Risk matrix

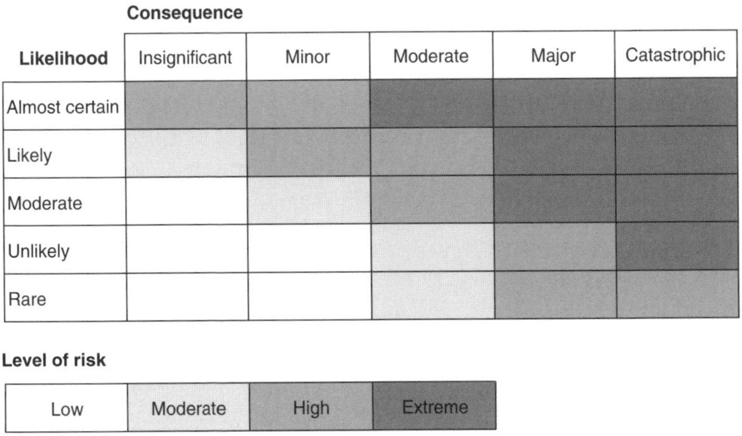

Consequence

Likelihood	Insignificant	Minor	Moderate	Major	Catastrophic
Almost certain					
Likely					
Moderate					
Unlikely					
Rare					

Level of risk

Low	Moderate	High	Extreme

Source: PRINCE2® Complete Document Templates Version 1.0 3/4/00 Rational Management Pty Ltd.

Verzuh describes various approaches to the issue of reducing project risk (1999:91–3):

- Accept the risk—that is, choose to do nothing about it.
- Avoid the risk—choose not to do part of the project.
- Monitor the risk and prepare contingency plans.
- Transfer the risk—for example, by taking out insurance.
- Mitigate the risk—in other words, 'work hard at reducing the risk'.

Once risks are understood, it is possible to identify contingencies—the 'what if' issues—and plan the response. Building and engineering projects always include a contingency allowance —money set aside for unforeseen circumstances, usually at about 10 per cent of the total cost. Projects in health and community services are often budgeted to the last penny, with no capacity for a contingency allowance. Even if adding an actual contingency allowance is not possible, there is usually a way to slip in some flexibility or some discretionary resources. When something goes wrong, perhaps resources allocated to another component of the project can be shifted without impacting on the core objectives, or there is some potential slack in the project timelines which can be taken up, or the scope can be squeezed by cutting back on non-core elements.

As part of contingency planning, it is important to plan for an escalation procedure. To 'escalate' means taking the project issue or issues higher in the organisation in order for them to be resolved, or implementing the next level of action identified to overcome an identified risk.

For more detailed guidance on risk management, see Australian standard AS/NZS 4360, available from Standards Australia (go to *http://www.standards.com.au/catalogue/ script/ search.asp*).

The quality plan

Every project aims to reach a standard of quality in its outcome— in order to be 'fit for purpose' at least, and perhaps to meet external standards (accreditation, ISO or other benchmarks) and to fit with the quality systems of the organisation. The project charter is again the source document for quality planning. What are the standards that each of the major deliverables or outcomes must meet? Are there process standards that apply (for example, 'consultation with unions is conducted in accordance with the organisation's formal agreements' or 'communication with staff is effective and conducted in accordance with the communication plan')? Who needs to be satisfied with the quality achieved?

Each project will have unique specifications, standards or criteria that need to be met. For example, a new information system might require an average response time of 3 seconds or less; a new strength and balance program for older people might have to achieve a high standard of safety. These requirements provide the elements for the project's quality plan. A simple quality plan for the emergency department project (introducing a new patient management system) is shown in Figure 9.

Figure 9: Quality plan for emergency department patient management system

Quality of outcomes	Measurement	Who assesses
The flow of patients through the department is efficient and safe	Meets specifications for timeliness and continuity of care	Directors (medical and nursing) of ED
The information needs of clinicians are met	Meets specifications; no losses of information currently available	Senior medical and nursing staff representatives
Administrative staff can meet their workloads with current staffing levels	Workload of new systems is at worst equal to existing	Administration manager
Process indicators		
Patient care is not disrupted during implementation	No adverse impact on patients is recorded during implementation	Directors of ED
Staff are consulted and engaged in changes affecting them	Meets organisational change agreement standards	Human resource consultant

Planning for variation

Projects never unfold exactly as planned, no matter how good the planning has been, and variations (or 'variances') are a normal part of project implementation. At the planning stage, it is important to anticipate the need for variations, and design a process for identifying, documenting and managing change. Formal tools for doing so are outlined below—they can be adapted to suit the needs of the project and the style of the organisation.

PRINCE and other frameworks call for a register of changes. Such a register would record a sequential numbering of each change, the problem/change title, originator, date notified, project manager approval data, sponsor or client approval date, implementation notes and, if relevant, change to the project completion date.

A register of issues is also suggested together with a protocol for management of those issues. During the course of the project, problems, situations, opportunities and errors can arise which are generally referred to as 'issues'; an issue can be defined as a problem or obstacle that the project team does not have the power to resolve (Verzuh 1999:230). Examples of issues could be delay in the supply of a project resource, unforeseen situations not dealt with in the project plan, a key stakeholder either leaving or joining the project, or software failure. As each issue is raised it is formally logged and thus has a place and a forum where actions can be assigned to the responsible person. The issue can then be tracked and given a priority to ensure that it is actioned at an appropriate time.

Figure 10: Contents of an issues log

Issue ID	Unique identifier, usually a number, assigned as each issue is identified.
Description	What is the issue and what is the impact if it is not resolved?
Assigned to	The project team member (or project manager) responsible for pursuing resolution.
Date identified	Date the issue was originally added to the log.
Current status/ last action	The date of the last action, a description of the action, and the current status of the issue. Leave all the action/status lines in the log as a record of how the action was pursued. Keeping closed issues in the log is one form of project history.

Source: Adapted from Verzuh (1999:230)

PLANNING PROJECT LOGISTICS

The project needs some systems under which to operate, and the physical resources to do so. The project plan should address the establishment logistics, the information systems and the methods for communication.

Project establishment logistics

To ensure a smooth start to project implementation, it's useful to plan the logistics for the establishment of the project. The following checklist highlights key issues:

- Is the project visible and identifiable; does it have a name or logo?
- Should the project be officially launched?
- Does the project have a home?
- Is there adequate space allocated for project team meetings, workspace for project staff, and for storage of project documents?
- Do you have the necessary resources, such as computers, access to photocopiers, fax machines, telephones and stationery? (A lot of time can be wasted in the early stages of project management in negotiating these basic things.)
- Is the project manager known and identified as being the project manager? Is the project manager the main or the only contact, and do people know how to make contact with the project?

The project information system

A vast array of information is generated during the life of a project. The documentation or data might include the project plan, training documentation, variation requests, progress and status reports, budget papers, scope documents, meeting minutes and agendas, Gantt and PERT charts or schedules, contracts, policies, feasibility studies, invoices and purchase orders, correspondence, workshop reports and so on.

Regardless of the size of your project, the plan should include a system for dealing with the data generated by it and with the information needed to manage it effectively. Early planning can also enable the learnings from the project to be held and shared more effectively across the organisation, and contribute to future project success.

Communications planning

Inevitably, almost all aspects of projects rely on effective communication—from policy decisions to meeting times. A breakdown in communication can be a project showstopper.

A communication plan is the written strategy for getting the right information to the right people at the right time (Verzuh 1999:67). All the project stakeholders will need information on a more or less regular basis, so even a simple plan outlining who requires the information, what information they need and when they need it is useful. A simple plan might look like the one outlined in Table 2.

Table 2: A simple communications plan

Stakeholder	Information required	Frequency	Medium
Sponsor	High level cost, quality, problems and proposed solutions	Monthly	Written report and meeting
Sponsor	Risk escalation	As necessary	Phone, email
Project team	Detailed schedule, problems, news, coordination information	Weekly	Meeting and status report
All interested parties	Occasional news of the project	As and when required	E-newsletter

In developing a communication plan it is useful to write a template for a status report that could be used for several stakeholders, so that progress can be communicated quickly and in a uniform manner. Also think about how reports and communication can be optimised for timeliness. Consider using paper reports, regular meetings, newsletters and message boards. A major project with multiple stakeholders might publish a newsletter, perhaps on the intranet, as illustrated by Case 12.

Case 12: The Friday Facts

The project manager for a multi-site project published a one- or two-page electronic update every Friday for 52 weeks—inevitably known as 'the Friday Facts'. It was sent to all interested people in five collaborating organisations spread over several cities and towns by email. The information was factual, the tone was casual and the layout was informal. Everyone who contributed was added to the email list, and the support staff appreciated being included and informed of the 'big picture'. For the recipients it was an easy way to keep up with the project, and it also contributed to overcoming the problems of distance in this complex project.

PLANNING FOR EVALUATION

The final component of the planning process is the evaluation plan, which essentially answers the question, 'Did the project achieve its goals?' Planning, implementing and evaluation are all part of an essentially cyclic activity where evaluation leads to another planning cycle in which you use what you have learned to improve the next project. When devising a plan it is wise to 'build in' the subsequent evaluation steps so that the evaluation starts while the program or project is actually running.

The project goal, objectives and sub-objectives provide the basis for the evaluation. The quality plan can also provide key elements. The evaluation plan should outline the standards, targets or outcomes against which the project will be measured, how the measurement will be made, and who will be involved. Chapter 7 addresses evaluation in more detail.

PLANNING FOR THE IRRATIONAL

We noted at the beginning of this chapter that reality hardly ever works out in the precise rational way that planning methods seem designed to achieve. This is not an argument against making a logical detailed plan, but it does point to the need for skilled management and flexibility.

Expecting the unexpected is the only possible outlook for project managers. In the next chapter we move to project management in action, and discuss how project teams manage what happens when the plan meets reality.

Postscript: The true story of medical emergency teams

The story of the establishment of a MET team developed in this chapter is not a true story, but MET teams are real, and this approach is becoming widespread. These teams enable hospitals to provide a much faster response to instability in vital signs and as a result to prevent some deaths. Rigorous evaluations have established that the death rate in at least some hospitals from 'critical events' can be reduced significantly through the use of a MET team. The MET approach also demonstrates that in some situations standard medical protocols, based on a long-established chain of command, are not the best method for managing care. It is important to note, however, that those same conventions protect quality of care in other important ways. As is often the case in quality stories, there is no one right answer, and the rightness of the answer changes over time.

SUMMARY

- Project planning is the critical success factor for projects and the project plan is the central pillar of project management.
- The rational planning approach involves the development of achievable aims, objectives and strategies in a logical order, even though reality hardly ever works that way.
- The foundation of the project plan is the project charter, which defines scope and strategies as well as aims and objectives.
- The other elements of the plan detail how the project charter will be implemented. They include the project structure, the work program and resources, planning for risk and quality, project logistics, and finally evaluation planning.
- Project committees and decision-making processes can be important methods of managing stakeholders, as well as coordinating the advice and inputs the project needs.
- If consumers will be affected by the project, there should be a method of engaging representatives in the project steering committee or other consultative mechanisms.
- The work program is the tasks and activities that will be undertaken and their schedule. Resources include the project team, specialist input and the budget.
- Risk management planning involves identifying what might go wrong, what will happen to the project if it does, how likely it is to happen, what contingency allowances can be made, and what approach to take to each major risk. The quality plan specifies the standards that the project's outcomes must meet, and how their achievement will be monitored.

- Project logistics include getting the project established (office, name, logo, etc.), the information systems the project will need and the communication plan.
- The plan should include a method of evaluating the success of the project.
- Even after writing a great plan, expect the unexpected.

6

IMPLEMENTATION PHASE: CARRYING OUT THE PLAN

'In strategy, the longest way round is often the shortest way home.'
(*Military historian Liddell Hart, quoted in Hilmer and Donaldson,
1996:x*)

The implementation (or execution) phase is when the rubber
hits the road for the project—when the long-planned actions are
taken, and strategies are implemented. When the project is under
way the project manager's focus shifts to two key goals: making
the project happen, and monitoring and measuring progress to
ensure that the project stays on track.

In this chapter we first discuss the management and leadership tasks of this phase, the skills of the project manager and some
techniques. Next we turn to the challenges of achieving change in
the project, and briefly outline some theories about change. We
suggest some methods for making change happen, and for
dealing with project politics and resistance to change. The final
section of the chapter addresses tasks, tools and techniques for
controlling and measuring the project's progress to successful
completion.

While in this chapter we differentiate the roles of the project
manager and the project team, we recognise that often a single
project officer takes on the functions of both manager and team,
frequently sharing the role of project manager with the person

they report to. They usually need to negotiate with other staff for contributions of time, energy and support, however. This is true for almost all projects in one way or another.

GETTING STARTED

Implementation of a project is about leading and motivating people, and coordinating human and other resources to carry out the plan. Controlling a project is about ensuring that its objectives are met by monitoring and measuring progress regularly to identify variances from the plan, and taking corrective action when it is needed (PMBOK 2000:30).

PMBOK (2000:35) describes the processes involved in the execution of a project as:

- Project plan execution—performing the activities on the plan.
- Quality assurance—evaluating the overall performance of the project to meet relevant quality standards.
- Team development—developing individual and group skills/competencies to enhance project performance.
- Information distribution—making needed information available to project stakeholders in a timely manner.

We would add to this list:

- Stakeholder management—working with stakeholders as the project unfolds, shoring up their commitment, responding to their concerns and monitoring any shifting alliances.

The sum total of these activities can be overwhelming for the project manager—so where do you start? The project plan is the key, and now is the time when the benefits of planning are seen. In cases where the project manager has been appointed after the development of the plan, a review of the plan is a good place to start. Is it realistic? Are there any glaring omissions? Was some of the planning not detailed enough? If there are problems with the plan at the commencement of project implementation, now is the time to address them—the sooner the better.

For a project manager new to the project and/or to the organisation or unit in which the project sits, the first step is to find out something about the project's history. How did it come about? Where did it develop? Is there someone in the senior management team who champions this project? If there is, does this person have a fixed view of how it should develop? Did someone else develop the project and expect to be its manager? If so, what is their attitude now, both towards the project team and the project?

Time spent on background at the beginning can help later on if the project seems to hit brick walls, or is being 'white anted', or when something is happening that you just cannot put your finger on. However, it is important not to be taken in by gossip (or to add to it), or to be seen to be 'taking sides' in broader disputes.

As the project is getting started, it's often a good idea to think about any sticking points that are likely to arise and how they could be resolved. This requires careful listening, honest thinking and informed logical analysis. It can be helpful to stand back from daily concerns and really analyse what's going on around the project and where the problems are likely to come from. One method is to tell yourself the story of how this project succeeds— what are the key mysteries that are solved, the lucky breaks, the turning points, that will make the difference? This technique can be used in the negative as well—if this project was to fail, what would the causes be, who would be the villains of the story? These techniques are a kind of rehearsal for managing and leading the project, and can be used in preparation for important presentations or meetings as well.

SKILLED PROJECT MANAGEMENT

'Project implementation is primarily about people. Only people can produce work and effort so your first concern must be how to lead and motivate your team.' (*Webster 1999:117*)

Achieving good project outcomes depends on good project management, and both the literature and all our interviewees stress the importance of having the right person or people to carry out this function. Project management is a set of methods but also an art. The art lies in understanding what the project must achieve, being constantly alert to contingencies and having the ability to be open and to respond in the right way— with flexibility, awareness of the situation and ability to deal with crises. Of equal importance are the ability to just get the job done and the persistence to keep the project moving on. As one of our interviewees put it, 'You need someone who keeps their eye on the ball, because projects need to be constantly worked and moved along in the right direction.'

There is a range of views about the importance of content knowledge for the project manager, that is, having expert knowledge in the area in which the project is being done. For example, in a project that will amalgamate two pathology services, how important is it that the project manager has a scientific background? For a project that will develop a service for newly-arrived immigrant women, does the project manager need a background in settlement work, and experience with the countries from which the women have come? How important are generic project management skills in these settings?

Our experience, and our research, indicate that content knowledge is a distinct advantage, and that a working familiarity with the culture of the organisation and the professional groups within it is almost essential. But project management skills are also essential. Our conclusion is that content knowledge should be defined fairly broadly. That is, for a project that will develop a new clinical service, knowing the clinical environment, its culture and dynamics is important, but you don't need to be an expert clinician. For an IT project, you need to understand the IT environment and information systems, but you don't have to be an expert programmer. On the other hand, where a potential project manager has great content knowledge and general management skills, but lacks project experience, some training, mentoring and support might bridge the gap.

When it comes to selection criteria and choosing the best person, the general principles for defining the required knowledge and skills for any job apply. Knowledge and skills should be specified in terms of the competence or ability required rather than particular qualifications or backgrounds. Careful definition of the requirements, so that there is a balance between strong content knowledge and project management ability, is also important.

All of these skills, attributes and knowledge add up to a tall order, and it must be said that much of what is required of a project manager is only gained through experience—of projects, of workplaces and of people. In our research, the managers generally felt that good project managers were rare, especially those with the skills to deal with complex or large projects. One commented that 'a good project manager is like gold and they're not very common'; another asserted that 'finding somebody who has real skills in that combination is rare'.

Respondents also thought that the softer or non-technical skills of project management, primarily the people (and political) skills, were of equal if not greater importance than technical project management skills: 'consulting, listening, working out the problems with the group . . . the process of project management is as important as the technical capability'.

Our respondents identified the following traits as being paramount for a project manager:

- Technical project management skills, know-how and capacity to 'do their homework'.
- Discipline and drive—application to the task, taking responsibility, decisiveness, ability to deal with detail.
- Vision and creative thinking—creating ownership, sharing the vision.
- Self-reflective—of their own practice, able to use judgment skills.
- Organised, with the ability to meet deadlines—follows up to ensure things are done.
- Initiative to work independently and 'pick up a project and run with it'.
- Communicative and articulate—talks to the right people, influences others, builds consensus, makes the project visible, negotiates, lobbies for the project.
- Analytical—keeps their eye on the ball, understands risk, can read situations.
- Flexible and open minded—able to deal with 'curve balls' and crises, actively solves problems and handles conflict.

Of course, no matter how experienced, competent, enthusiastic and intelligent the person chosen for the job of project manager may be, they cannot expect to operate effectively without support and cooperation from senior management, staff engaged in the project and the organisation at large (Lock 2001). Good project managers are not made or developed overnight. However, experienced line managers will already have many of the skills and attributes outlined above, and the skills of project management can be learnt (see, for example, some of the resources listed in Chapter 3).

We saw some evidence that the strategy of developing promising project staff internally has greater long-term benefits than the option of buying in project management skills. Some of the organisations we studied had taken a long-term view, and had worked to develop a 'project management culture' or to encourage project thinking throughout their organisations. They also invested in both formal training and informal learning opportunities for key members of their staff.

Leadership, motivation and teamwork

The project management literature, our informants and our own experience tell us that leadership, motivation and teamwork are essential in creating successful project outcomes. When people speak of leadership they suggest clear vision, good people skills and good process skills are essential; when they speak of motivation they suggest that building commitment and creativity are essential. When we think of teamwork we think of interpersonal skills, working well in groups and working to a common purpose. The guidelines in the box below can help project managers achieve these objectives.

Leadership and teamwork guidelines for the project manager

- Do not lose sight of the aim of the project—whatever strategies you develop they must be focused on achieving the aim.
- Timelines are important—while some flexibility might be necessary too much flexibility will see you lose control of the project.
- Problems and potential problems must be identified and dealt with—they will not go away, and might get bigger and come back to bite you at the most inconvenient time.
- Attention to detail is essential—it can help you identify problems and keep your eye on emerging issues, so keep good notes and records.
- Keep your eye on the ball—work the project; it will not happen by itself.
- Walk your talk—make sure that you do what you say you will do; model good project management practice.

- Hone your communication skills—Are you a good listener? Are you approachable? Provide clear, easy-to-read written reports and memos that are short and to the point.
- Improve your facilitation skills, especially in meetings —make all meetings productive or people will stop attending.
- Recognise the skills of others, praise where appropriate, notice the work of others—give credit where credit is due.
- Take responsibility—beware of blaming others for problems.
- Encourage good working relationships—through good humour, a positive attitude and a 'can do' approach.
- Aim to be someone who creates and gives out good energy—not a black hole who sucks the energy out of others.

One of the more challenging leadership tasks in project teams is to ensure that the team constantly assesses and refines the project's methods and focus, in response to either changes in the project's environment, or a growing knowledge of what will really enable the project idea to work in practice. Action learning (or the related idea of reflective practice) is an approach which may be useful for this task. Action learning is the act of thoughtful consideration (and discussion) of events, a process by which project participants make sense of their experience, and its meaning (DeFilippi 2001).

Project managers can promote action learning in their teams by the simple method of encouraging thoughtful discussion and analysis of any aspect of a project which seems either troublesome or potentially rewarding. Regular team meetings could be used both to address normal project business and to encourage reflection and learning. The major challenge with this technique is to establish an environment of trust and safety for team members to engage in open, thoughtful discussion; and then to maintain a climate of safety through mutual commitment to confidentiality and constructive use of the discussion outcomes.

Managing project staff

Building a team that works well together is a key part of project success. All the normal requirements of good people management and effective teamwork apply. Good management of a project team also requires effective responses to three important considerations.

First, team members will probably only report to the project manager for the duration of the project, or may continue to be supervised by their normal line manager throughout. In this situation, loyalty to the manager and the project needs a basis other than long-term mutual interest or dependence. Openness between the two managers involved can help avoid a situation where the team member feels pulled in two directions. A clear delineation of the split in reporting relationships is essential— for example: Who approves leave? Who does performance appraisal? Who can make demands on the person's time and for what? What are the confidentiality expectations?

Second, team members may have only some of the skills the project needs, but the project cannot wait for long-term skill development. In this case, training workshops might be held in order to finalise the project's chosen methods, tools, templates and reports, and to train team members in their use. Other topics, such as running effective meetings, process mapping techniques, interviewing skills and so on, could also be covered. Skill levels can improve rapidly when tools and templates are used consistently across the team, and team members are able to use the project manager and other leaders as models. Staff should be given the opportunity to identify their areas of interest and strength as well as those areas where they lack skills or confidence. Then either their roles can be structured accordingly, or further skills training can be arranged.

While it is not possible for the project to take a long-term view, the organisation needs to. The development of a cadre of skilled project staff and future project leaders can be a real strategic advantage arising from small investments consistently made, project by project. The appointment of experienced project managers as mentors can also add significantly to the capability and future development of project staff.

Finally, towards the end of the project, there will be a tendency for team members (and maybe the manager) to look around, focusing on returning to their units or getting their next job rather than on finishing the project (Young 1997:135). It is a good idea to raise this issue at the beginning and work out strategies for meeting both the needs of the team members and the needs of the project. Team members may be inclined to deny that this is an issue—particularly if the team climate is not supportive. If everyone denies the existence of the issue it may be that the team has two problems, not one (a climate that is not seen as safe, and a potential problem with retention of staff), and the manager needs to work on both.

At least the manager, and maybe one or two others, could be contracted until well after the expected completion date to allow for slippage and for finishing and bedding-down activities. This will give them a period after the project is practically completed to focus on their next moves. Team members and the project manager could also negotiate agreements with the home base manager to cover problems with timing or any other aspect of the return to home base, and a process to be followed if these contingencies arise.

Early attention to these important issues, and establishing an environment of safety and clear expectations among the project team, will pay off in enhanced capacity to deliver results, and to weather storms, as the project progresses.

Problem-solving skills

During the course of the project it might become obvious that the project team has gaps in its skills and knowledge, or conflicts might emerge between team members or other groups and individuals. This can be one of the most challenging things that a manager has to deal with, inside or outside a project. While there are many techniques and methods for dealing with conflict, basic problem-solving skills are particularly relevant.

It is important to keep an open mind to allow you to recognise problems as they begin to emerge in the project team. Webster (1999) suggests the following problem-solving process:

■   Accept that a problem exists and resolve to take action.
■   Dispassionately gather the facts.
■   Define the problem.
■   Understand what is causing the problem.
■   Engage the team in contributing to both understanding the problem and finding solutions.
■   Plan the response and implement it.

Conducting effective meetings

Project meetings fulfil many important functions in most projects, and are necessary for effective communication. They will be more effective if they are properly scheduled, have a well-structured agenda, and are briefly recorded in minutes that include required action. There will be different types of meetings with different people participating—project team, steering committee, executive briefings, stakeholder meetings—which will probably require different approaches to decision making, structuring the agenda, facilitating discussion and reporting progress and outcomes.

Good meeting and facilitation skills can help to save time, diffuse conflict and make things happen. There are two underlying principles in facilitation. The first is the need to be efficient—people are busy and hate to waste valuable time in unproductive meetings. The second is participation—people need to have their voices heard and feel that they are contributing if they are to have some ownership of the project and maintain their commitment. We suggest the following guidelines for good facilitation.

Guidelines for effective project meetings

- Always have an agenda—no matter how small and informal the meeting.
- Know the meeting timelines and stick to them—put time limits against agenda items and stick to them unless there is a very good reason not to.
- The facilitator does not have to know the answer to every question—put difficult points back to the meeting.
- Keep things moving along—do not let participants ramble.
- Encourage some people to speak.
- Be prepared to shut others up—nicely!
- Keep on track—don't be taken off into irrelevant issues.
- Look for answers to difficult problems.
- Make sure every issue has an action—even if it is just 'leave to next meeting'.
- Make sure each action has someone who is responsible for making it happen.
- Keep notes or minutes.
- Make sure you revisit them at the next meeting and deal with any matters arising.
- Keep a record of attendance.

USING THE PROJECT TO ACHIEVE CHANGE

We turn now to the major implementation challenge the project team will face—achieving change through the project. A clinician manager we interviewed in a major teaching hospital was emphatic about the central role of change in projects in his organisation: 'Projects are one of the biggest single enablers of changing the way we do things, a way of bringing more people on board to be part of the solution and adapt to the kind of emerging changes that seem to grow in number every year. The objective is to shift the way things are done.' Another manager believed that change is the defining feature of a project: 'projects are about changing the way people do things'. And virtually all of our respondents saw the problem of resistance to change as a key driver of project failure.

Usually the whole purpose of a project is to bring in something new or to do something differently—that is, to innovate. Innovation is defined as the successful implementation of something new, or more simply, as 'putting ideas to work' (Department of Industry, Science and Resources 2000:9). In health and community services, as in other spheres, innovation happens when a new process or system is introduced, even if the agency is not the first in the world to undertake that particular change. This definition recognises that a real but sometimes neglected challenge in innovation lies not so much in knowing the right answer, as in achieving the changes necessary to have it adopted (Dwyer and Leggat 2002).

In this section we focus on projects which need to achieve change in some aspect of the existing work system, power structure, working relationships, roles or responsibilities of people and teams—that is, where the change will affect people and their work. A lot has been written about achieving change in organisations, and much of it applies to projects. We first briefly review some of the major theories and approaches to change that are relevant to project management and the politics of change, and then address the ways people respond to change and the central theme of resistance. There is only a small body of research on the project management of organisational change. Most of the research focuses on the technical aspects of project management and the successful management of individual projects (Partington 1996), and presents a rational approach to change in project management processes, emphasising the importance of goals, planning, tasks, staff, tools, timelines and resources but ignoring the people side of change. Yet our research indicates that it is more often the people side of project management than any other single factor that leads to project failure.

Participative approaches to implementing change

The organisational change theorists tell us that while directive processes can achieve change quickly, it is the more participative approaches to change that create a sense of ownership and involvement of the major players. For example, research from the UK and New Zealand (Perkins et al. 1997) demonstrates that senior medical staff are more likely to support change when they have had some involvement in the decision-making processes. The main critiques of participative change processes, such as organisational development, are the slow pace of change in small incremental steps, failure to deal with the difficulties in participation, and lack of acknowledgment of issues of power.

The change that is part of a project is by its very nature proactive change, although the project may have originated as a response to an external event or crisis. Projects are also generally aimed at sustainable change—making sure that something not only changes in the short term but also becomes a feature of organisational practice. Both of these characteristics tend to argue for a participative approach.

McElroy (1996) articulates a clear argument in favour of the use of projects for achieving organisational change. He contrasts four methods of implementing change:

- education and communication (persuading staff of the need);
- participation (staff assist management to define the change and the change process);
- intervention (management defines the required outcomes but uses projects to enable participation in the process); and
- edict (where management gives precise instructions to be followed),

and concludes that intervention—that is, management of change by projects—is the form most certain of success.

One of the problems in the health and community services sector is that much of the change that has taken place over the past few years has been radical, top down, directive change as organisations have had to respond quickly to budget cuts, policy directives and shifting government priorities. Strategies that Kotter and Schlesinger (1979) describe as manipulation, co-option, and explicit and implicit coercion have been used. But, as many managers have found, there are problems with these strategies in the human services industry, and in any case they are most often not available to project managers.

Change makers: the surgeon, the scientist, the nurse and the administrator

There are many approaches to change not recommended in the management literature. These are some that can be observed on field trips:

- The surgeon: Make the decision and do it. Just do it. The crash or crash through approach.
- The scientist: Get the right answer. Verify the data and the logic. Then it will just happen—won't it?
- The nurse: Look over there! See, it didn't hurt a bit, did it? The distraction method.
- The administrator: Process, process, process. Change by exhaustion.

Each of these can work for some things sometimes. But there are better ways.

Managing participation

We advocate the use of participatory methods to engage staff and stakeholders and enhance the momentum of the project. But there is also the 'tyranny of participation' or 'death by process'— endless meetings, surveys, workshops and interim reports. The challenge is to balance openness, transparency and consultation with actually moving forward, while also avoiding the 'crash through or crash' approach.

There are two elements to managing participation. One is the project's leadership structure, including the engagement of stake-holders in committees, and we have discussed this in Chapter 5 and elsewhere in this chapter. The second is broader participation by staff generally and by members of stakeholder groups. The key to success with these methods is structured participation, with well-designed processes that ask the right questions at the right stage, and recognise that people want to have their say, but are also busy.

The most effective participation processes use a range of methods tailored to the needs of the project, the participants and the style of the organisation. They pose questions for debate and solutions that are relevant to the participants, that will be genuinely useful to the project and are held at the right time in the project's life. They make the givens explicit, such as decisions already made by the executive or board, or the implications of government policy or legislation, to provide a framework around the areas of discretion. And they do not ask people to start with a blank canvas if this is not the real situation.

For some people being able to make a submission is important. Alternatively, when the project team needs to understand the thinking of particular groups, confidential one-to-one or small group discussions with project staff, or others who are trusted by the group, might be the only effective method. This approach can enable the project team to get the insights it needs and lets the relevant group see that their views are taken seriously. Safeguards to protect the rights and interests of line managers can be built in to this process, so it doesn't become either a witch-hunt or a method of undermining the effectiveness of management.

For some questions, straw polls or 'dotmocracy' (see Case 6 in Chapter 4) can produce surprising results that capture the majority view more accurately than open discussion which may be dominated by particular individuals. Computer-based voting systems have the advantage of allowing instant collation of results and producing graphs which clearly demonstrate the balance of views. The disadvantages of these systems are cost and the logistics of setting them up. Sometimes a conflicted group will agree that the project should consult an independent expert and will accept that person's opinion on particular issues.

The general principle is to use appropriate methods to gather meaningful results with an explicit method of analysing and using the outcomes. Most importantly, there needs to be a method of closing off the participation exercise and moving on. For further information about how to manage participation, skilled workshop facilitators are recommended.

The politics of change: managing the shadow side

In any discussion of organisational change, the issues raised are often essentially 'political'. By political we mean the methods by which people seek, acquire and use power (Pinto 2000:85). This brings in the power structure and relationships, and the tactics and strategies people use to enhance their power or their access to prized resources. It also includes the alliances and groupings that share and use power and influence, and the resources, information and support on which they are built.

One of the reasons that many change processes fail is that the proponents do not understand the politics of change. The health and community services sector is comprised of many powerful stakeholders who do not always have the same interests and often compete with each other for power and prestige. Organisations survive in an environment of contradiction and conflict, managing tensions between providing a service and balancing a budget, between their espoused policy and their actual practice, between centralism and localism, between professionals and managers and between change versus tradition and comfort.

Managing change is a political process, and some writers argue that the ability to achieve change is a function of power and influence rather than method (Stephenson 1985). For Nadler and Tushman (1997), change management is a problem of power, of anxiety, and of organisational control. The response should be shaping political behaviour, motivating constructive behaviour and managing the transition.

While some of the elements of the power structure (like formal hierarchies, controls and resource allocation) are overt, much of the politics of the organisation, and of the project, happen in what Egan (1994) calls the 'shadow side'. The shadow side is

> all the important activities and arrangements that do not get identified, discussed, and managed in decision-making forums that can make a difference. The shadow side deals with the covert, the undiscussed, the undiscussable and the unmentionable. It includes arrangements not found in organisational manuals and company documents or on organisational charts (Egan 1994:4).

The shadow side is outside ordinary managerial intervention and can substantially affect productivity and the quality of working life, both positively and negatively. A supportive organisational culture is a powerful positive element of the shadow side. Other positive aspects include informal advocacy on behalf of the organisation which many staff undertake both in and outside of work settings, and informal networks of communication that flow under and around formal channels and help both managers and staff know what is going on. Negative elements can include things like entrenched enmity between functional managers (affecting the ability of their departments to work together) and a culture that accepts poor performance by favoured individuals. Another kind of negative element occurs when a board member is influenced in their decision making by loyalty to an outside force rather than the best interests of the organisation itself.

There will always be a shadow side, and organisations will always have politics. The question is not whether, but how much and in what directions (helpful or harmful to the agency). Good management, tolerance of difference and debate, and open communication will tend to minimise the space that the shadow side has to work in. That is, bringing important issues into the open and dealing with them in a careful way will reduce the need for shadow-side activity. Projects can be an ideal opportunity to shine the spotlight on forgotten cupboards and remote attics in the organisation and to deal constructively with shadow-side issues.

There are many managers, and project managers, who feel that politics is a dirty business, and would like to see themselves as operating above or outside it. Politics can indeed be unpleasant, but staying outside is really not possible. Dealing ethically with organisational politics, and your own role within them, requires skill and strategy. The first skill is the ability to see and 'read' what is going on. The second is to know how to challenge the negatives creatively. The third is to be able to turn discomfort and disruption into learning.

Project managers by and large do not have a strong or stable power base (Pinto 2000), and must learn to cultivate influence instead. This need is exacerbated by the fact that projects often exist outside the traditional functional structure and so all resources must be negotiated and bargained for. Lack of authority, for example, to conduct a performance review of project team members, also limits power, and project managers may even be managing their peers or their superiors. They have little managerial control in this situation and so human skills become very important. As Pinto (2000:86) argues, 'successful project managers are those who intuitively understand that their job consists of more than simply being technically and managerially competent'.

This has many implications for project politics. Pinto identifies a number of key issues. The first is that project managers must understand and acknowledge the political nature of most organisations, especially the influence of key stakeholders. The second is that project managers must learn to cultivate 'appropriate' political tactics.

One important tactic is to use the 'WIIFM' principle—what's in it for me? That is, departmental or unit loyalties and interests are usually more immediate and more powerful than commitment to organisation-wide concerns. The project manager can benefit by analysing proposals and issues from the point of view of each of the departments whose contribution, or acquiescence, is needed. When people respond to a proposal by asking 'What's in it for me?', they are offering an opportunity for the project manager to explain why they should support the project. Power can be also enhanced through tactics that level the playing field, like establishing a superior knowledge base and using it to add value (Pinto 2000).

Stephenson (1990) argues that the necessary skills include negotiating and bargaining, urging and cajoling and coping with resistance. He also suggests assessing the power of opposing forces, forming coalitions and choosing optimal timing for action. In real life, the champions of change juggle opportunities, problems, the shadow side of the organisation and their upward management issues, and a combination of good luck, good ideas and good management gets them through. Whatever model or strategy for change management is used, the 'pointy end' of change management in projects is dealing with the response typically labelled 'resistance'. We use this label in the following sections, but it's important to note that some of what is called resistance to change is motivated by concern about technical errors or wrong-headed policies. A lot of this concern can be met with a listening ear, and improvements to project design can result—not all resistance is motivated by self-interest, nor is it necessarily a threat to the project.

The rationale of resistance

When changes are proposed, the people who will be affected begin calculating gains and losses in relation to two basic questions: What's in it for me? Will it really happen? There are some good reasons for the tendency to resist change. Those who are comfortable with the way things are will often see, perhaps correctly, that they have something to lose, including some of the power or influence they currently hold in their teams or in the wider organisation or field. And they will often have some power which they can use to resist, as Case 13 illustrates.

Case 13: Understanding resistance to change

The consulting doctors whose lives are organised within a complex web of sessional arrangements and a daily round of attendances at several hospitals have good practical reasons to resist a proposal for daily morning ward rounds in one of the hospitals in which they work. And the reasons persist even if payment for their time is adequate, and regardless of how much more efficient it might make the care of their patients in that hospital. They also have the power of their independence and often the market (that is, they will be hard to replace). Gnashing of managerial teeth, and exhortations to 'think of the greater good', are unlikely to be very persuasive. For change to happen, the consultants' real difficulties and best interests are going to have to be understood and responded to, as the power of the manager to force change is probably limited.

On the other hand, those who stand to gain from a proposed change, either personally or because they agree with the goals of the change, are in a position of uncertainty. Their active support generally depends not only on whether they can see that there is something in it for them, but also on whether they believe it will really happen.

Resistance can occur anywhere. Individuals and groups without strong power find ways to resist change, and senior managers whose areas are affected by the project might also use tactics of resistance. Some of the direct and indirect approaches to resistance are summarised below (with apologies to the animal world).

Changing resistance

Perhaps one of the most famous models of change is Lewin's force field analysis. Lewin (1958) sees the change process as a struggle

The art of resistance

There are many ways of resisting change if you don't want it to happen. These are some of the tried and true methods:

- The White Ant: Sneaks around pointing out all the possible downsides, no matter how far-fetched or unlikely. 'If you go to daylight saving, the cream will curdle and the scones won't rise.' Undermines and actively works against change.
- The Beaver: Mobilises resentment about every problem, and every change in living memory, to build a dam of resistance. 'You could let them know how angry you are about the new intake system by helping me to stop them from changing the team structure, and anyway, we haven't recovered from the millennium bug yet.'
- The Tortoise: Never comes to meetings about proposals he doesn't like the sound of, and doesn't read emails advising how to contribute; moves slowly on everything related to the proposal, and grumbles quietly in the tearoom about not being consulted. 'Don't talk to me, don't change anything without talking to me, and don't move so fast.'
- The Kangaroo: Usually a senior manager, hops from one idea to the next, and appears just before sunset wanting to change the project scope. 'You've built a great battleship, now let's make it fly.'
- The Red Herring: Finds a very interesting distraction to complicate and bedevil the path of the project. 'The new filing system will be great, but only if we can reorganise the Christmas holiday roster by Friday.'

between the driving forces for change and the restraining forces for maintaining the status quo, as represented in Figure 11. According to Lewin's model, the change agent should first of all identify through qualitative research the forces for and the forces against the change. An assessment can then be made as to which

Figure 11: Force field analysis

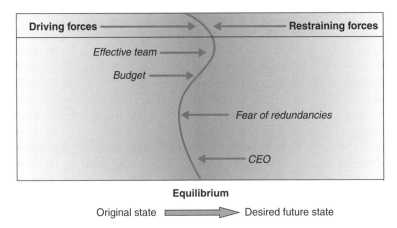

Source: Martin and Henderson (2001:128)

of the forces are strongest and weakest, and what strategies are needed to support the positives and weaken the negatives. In Figure 11, the project is championed by a senior manager, and supported by an effective confident team (which needs to be sustained through the change process) and a budget imperative. The change could affect staffing numbers, so fear of redundancies is a force of resistance. The senior manager also knows that although the CEO professes support, she will be watching to ensure that the senior manager is kept in line. The senior manager believes this problem can be headed off, so the CEO is therefore listed as a weak force of resistance.

Martin and Henderson (2001) also point out that 'pull' tactics as well as 'push' can be used to move the line of resistance— sometimes it is more effective to focus on weakening resistance than on strengthening the forces for change. For example, the fear of redundancies will not go away because positive forces are strengthened. It is more effectively dealt with directly, by providing cast-iron assurances (if there really will be no redundancies) or by negotiating principles for protecting the interests of staff (if redundancies are on the cards). On the other hand, the weak potential for problems with the CEO is best dealt with indirectly through strengthening the positives of trust and accountability in the manager's relationship with the CEO.

151

The next stage is to unfreeze patterns of behaviour on three levels—the individual level, the level of structures and systems and the organisational climate/interpersonal level. Unfreezing patterns of behaviour at each level is intended to make them responsive to change by unblocking existing systems. This is followed by the stage of movement or transition, followed by the refreezing of the new patterns of behaviour or the institutionalisation of change. Lewin recognised that the intervening transition requires careful management and thoughtful implementation tactics.

The value of Lewin's model is that it can be applied to almost any change situation. It provides a way of identifying the hidden forces that can derail the change process and the analytical basis for a strategy for dealing with them. Like the stakeholder analysis map in Chapter 5 (Figure 4), it can help the project manager to identify the important resistors that need to be removed, and the important supporters that need to be nurtured and mobilised.

As noted above, there are always good reasons for resistance. Tactics for reducing or removing resistance are generally based on an understanding of the needs and interests of the groups involved. For project managers there are two basic routes: buy them off or change their hearts and minds, or both. It may be possible, for example, to move the positions of some of the players on the field so that interests are realigned, or to convince them that change is needed through well-presented data and analysis. For some people, being brought into the tent (that is, included on committees or in formal and informal meetings) will be enough to move them from mild resistance to open-minded monitoring or even a position of support.

Listening to resistance

'Strategically, we should belittle our enemies, but technically, we should take them very seriously.' (*Mao Zedong*)

It is also likely that at least some of the resistance will be well informed and well intentioned. Understanding and analysing the sources of resistance will often lead to change in the project— for example, staff members' concern about the costs of change may be based on a more detailed understanding of current reality than the project manager enjoys. Each issue must be judged objectively on its merits. Resistance to change is not always a bad thing, as Kahn (1982:416) argues:

> In considering obstacles to change, we must keep in mind the deceptive nature of our concepts. When we want change, we speak of those who do not as presenting obstacles and resistance. When we want stability, we speak of perseverance and commitment among those who share our views. The behavior of people in the two situations may be identical; it is their stance relative to our own that dictates our choice of language.

When project changes are made in response to feedback from stakeholders, the situation should be presented openly and with appreciation, as illustrated by Case 14. It is the project manager's responsibility to follow through with any needed adjustments to the project plan, including its timetable or strategies.

Case 14: Change and chest pain

A project which aimed to establish a chest pain evaluation unit in a hospital emergency department was commenced with great enthusiasm and a reasonable amount of funding. These units accept patients who might have heart problems, and provide fast, specialised assessment within the emergency setting. Only about one-third of all patients with chest pain need admission to hospital, so this service enables those who need cardiac care to get it quickly, while those whose pain has a different cause can be identified quickly and treated, usually without admission. It is a good model, with a lot of benefits to all categories of patients.

However, implementing such a unit in a large teaching hospital required emergency department staff, cardiologists, technical and diagnostic staff to work differently, and there was initially much suspicion about whose turf was being invaded and who would have to work harder. The project manager and the executive in charge of the area recognised an emerging risk, and acted to bring these powerful stakeholders together. A working party was established in which a representative of each major group was asked to contribute to an analysis of the changes in work flow, need for inpatient beds, revenue generation, record keeping, equipment needs and so on. The legitimate interests of each stakeholder were heard and respected, and solutions to pressure points (such as the management of patients between midnight and 6 am) were carefully developed. The project broadened its focus from clinical protocols and space requirements to a comprehensive assessment of the impact of actual and potential changes.

Project bureaucracy and organisational change: a paradox

We have argued throughout this book that project management is all about change. But there are two paradoxes that should be noted. The first is that an over-bureaucratic model of project management might actually impede organisational change (Partington 1996). Emphasis on rigid control through adherence to detailed plans and budgets and tight timelines can work against the emerging, iterative nature of many change projects in health and community services. The real solutions to problems in models of care or support systems are often not known at the beginning of a project, which may be why a project approach to the problem has been chosen. In this case, the project team and the stakeholders need to be flexible in their expectations of exactly what will emerge at the other end, how and when. The project plan is still a vital component, but the need to plan for variation is also a strong one. Project managers must avoid falling in love with their plans.

The second paradox is the fact that senior managers may, in effect, be asked to disempower themselves and at the same time impose more discipline on themselves (Partington 1996). Partington points out that the organisational change literature argues that the support of top management is essential if change is to be realised, yet in practice there is tension between project-based authority (held by the project manager) and the functional authority of line managers. As Partington notes, 'it is natural for managers at every level to struggle against the abandonment of hierarchies' (1996:18). Some of the organisations we studied experienced problems with ownership or buy-in during the project as a result of the struggle to protect power, and transferability or sustainability of the outcomes after completion of the project also suffered.

Projects may also effectively ask managers to exercise their authority differently, and with more discipline. By locking managers as well as staff into specified goals, strategies, outcomes and budgets, projects can be seen as a temporary and partial stay on the ability of senior managers to change their minds and manage separate parts of their operations separately and incrementally. In some cases the leadership level may not have project expertise, and may lack the skills to operate competently in a project environment—for example, not knowing how to respond to the challenges of managing a matrix of projects and line operations (Partington, 1996).

The solution to this second problem is a long-term one which must be tackled by the organisation as a whole. However, the project manager who is aware of these issues can at least understand some of the sources of resistance from above, and at best can design ways of working around them.

CONTROL AND MONITORING DURING IMPLEMENTATION

So far, we have discussed the challenges of making projects, and particularly organisational change, happen. In the rest of this chapter we turn to some of the tools and techniques that assist project managers to maintain control and monitor the progress of projects through to successful completion. The separation between these two goals is a little artificial—control and monitoring play a key role in making the project happen; and the effectiveness of implementation can either support or challenge control and effective monitoring.

Some organisations have mandated methods that they use for control and monitoring of projects. However, for most of the organisations we studied there was either no mandated method, or there was a lot of flexibility about mixing and matching tools according to the needs of the project.

Methods and tools are important for control and monitoring, and decisions should be made as early as possible about which ones will be used. You may need to import or develop your own templates, forms, data collection and reporting processes. The challenge might be the adaptation of tools and methods to the more difficult realm of organisational change projects. We discuss several of the available methods in the rest of this chapter.

Webster (1999) suggests that three types of information are required to control a project—historical, present (diagnostic) and future (prognostic)—and that information for a good control system should be visible, accurate, reliable, valid, timely and prognostic. To determine what information about project progress or performance needs to be collected, monitored and reported during the life of the project, consult the project plan. The plan should contain all the project parameters that require monitoring, and hence enable the design of a monitoring system. What needs to be monitored relies heavily on the nature of the project—however, it is likely that data on expenditure (compared to budget), task/activity completion (compared to the schedule) and performance data (compared to specifications) will be monitored. Meredith and Mantel (2000) suggest that while it is easy to focus on monitoring data that is easily gathered, monitoring should concentrate primarily on measuring important facets of output (for example, the extent to which system design has been completed), rather than on intensity of activity (for example, the number of meetings that have been held) (Meredith and Mantel 2000:414–15).

There are several aspects of any project that will require project management skills for monitoring and controlling. We briefly address controlling the scope and schedule, the budget and resources, project quality, risk and contingencies, before turning to the challenge of managing projects when they get into trouble.

Keeping to the plan

'Project plans are not very useful if no one follows them. Successful project managers establish ways to ensure that their projects proceed according to plans.' (*Kliem et al. 1997:202*)

Having ensured that the project is well planned and scoped, the role of the project manager is then to ensure that the project progresses smoothly according to the project plan (unless variations are agreed—see later in this chapter). The amount and quality of project planning will quickly become evident in the implementation phase. Any deficiency of planning may not be the project manager's doing, as not all project managers have the benefit of being involved in the project from the beginning, but the project manager is the one who will deal with the consequences.

It should also be noted that the tasks of planning, monitoring and controlling are cyclical—that is, the cycle of planning, checking on progress, comparing progress to the plan and taking corrective action if progress does not match the plan is followed by another round of planning to incorporate any necessary changes (Meredith and Mantel 2000:412).

The general methods for monitoring adherence to project plans are status collection and assessment against the baseline provided by the plan, and perhaps by other sources. These methods involve collecting defined information to measure the progress of both the entire project and the activities within it (Kliem et al. 1997:202). The multitude of ways of gathering data and information on what is actually happening in the project range from the 'corridor chat' to the reports generated by an information system; for example, a financial report showing actual costs versus the budget. When the data generated are meaningful and reasonably accurate, the information can be a powerful impetus towards goal attainment—achieving milestones and outcomes—for teams and stakeholders.

Controlling project scope and the schedule

The chart or graphical display is both the most common and the simplest way to represent data in order to monitor and control a project. A bar or line graph can easily show progress in each aspect of a project compared to the project plan. Virtually any aspect of a project can be measured, and the priority is to chart the critical factors for project success. Examples of the items that are often charted in this way include:

- project task progress (percentage completion of project tasks as a whole by week);
- staff utilisation (for example, percentage usage by week);
- performance (for example number and magnitude of variations);
- task hours and percentage complete; and
- customer satisfaction measures or milestones.

For projects that are structured in stages, the finishing of one stage, sign-off and commencement of the next, are another opportunity for controlling the scope and schedule. At the commencement of the new stage, progress and the potential for variations can be reviewed, as demonstrated in Case 15.

Case 15: Preparing for Y2K

As it turned out the night was a fizzer—even the hospital emergency departments were unusually quiet. But a senior IT manager, looking back on all the preparation, felt that it had been worth it. 'The risk analysis was a great learning experience, and we had a much better understanding of where we needed to focus the development and replacement effort for our systems. There is now a much higher general level of awareness in the sector about the need for contingency planning and preparedness. One of the techniques we used, to try and maintain some sense of control in what was a really pressured lead-up to the big night, was charting progress visually against a long list of actions required to prevent, avoid and manage the risks, and implement contingency arrangements.'

Figure 12 shows a small section of the master chart.

Figure 12: Monitoring progess

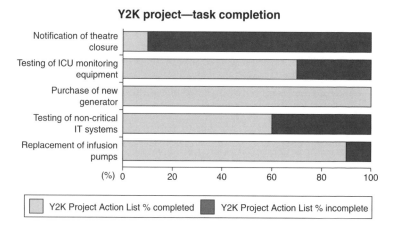

Y2K project—task completion

Y2K Project Action List % completed   Y2K Project Action List % incomplete

Controlling the budget and resources

The budgeting and estimation of project costs is difficult and often poorly done, which can mean in turn that it is difficult to control the costs of a project against the plan. Also, if the budget is not altered when the scope of a project changes, there is little chance that the costs will match it.

Monitoring of actual and forecast expenditure against budget is probably one of the most familiar control tools in the management tool kit. Good information is an important aid to the control of costs, but in the end hard decisions may be required. As noted in Chapter 5, there are several kinds of contingency response that might be called on—finding other sources of funding, reducing the scope, taking up slack in one part of the project to support another part's shortfall, or moving team members around to meet priority needs.

Managing quality

Quality and safety are vital in health and community services, and this applies to projects as much as to ongoing service delivery. There is often a short chain between a project and the direct implications for the care and safety of patients or clients.

When projects are in the implementation phase, the pressure to cut corners in order to maintain progress may be significant. If performance criteria have been defined in the planning phase (see the quality planning section in Chapter 5), the focus during implementation is firstly to ensure that they are made explicit and understood by all stakeholders. This is one of the reasons why it is a good idea to set up quality assurance mechanisms which are transparent and require reporting to the sponsor or project steering committee on a regular basis.

The second focus of quality monitoring is to ensure that any variation from the quality plan is logged, documented and resolved at a high level. A procedure for acceptance of variations from the quality plan should be formalised (usually either through the project steering committee or the customer or sponsor).

Some project teams appoint a 'quality partner'—a friendly expert adviser who takes a watching brief, not waiting for the documentation of problems, but working confidentially with team to prevent them. An experienced project manager or a person with expertise in quality in the relevant area could play this role.

Managing risk and contingency

During the implementation phase in any project, changes to the plan (or 'variances' or 'variations') are normal and to be expected. If there are significant variances (and they jeopardise the project objectives), the plan can be adjusted by repeating the relevant planning process—for example, re-estimating staffing levels (PMBOK 2000).

Change is a healthy part of project life, and is to be expected, but it needs to be controlled (Healy 1997:256). It is inevitable that as soon as the project plan and scope have been written and agreed to, changes will occur. The important issue for control is to ensure that variances are documented, the plan is adjusted accordingly, and the variance is formally accepted by the authorised group or individual.

Project management offers some excellent methods and techniques for controlling the activities in the implementation phase to assist in ensuring that the project doesn't go off the rails (that is, result in an outcome that was not planned for). Whether or not some of these events are significant, are acceptable or indeed are welcomed, depends largely on the project itself and the organisation.

When the project is being conducted by external consultants, the contract will usually include a provision for variations. This protects the consultant from escalating costs due either to fickle decision making by the client or to genuine contingencies arising in the project, things not reasonably foreseen. The contract will also usually contain clauses that enable the client to extract additional work if the variation is of the consultant's making (for example, poor modelling) or to reduce or withhold payments if the quality standards are not met.

The best outcome for a troubled project may in fact be to terminate it before further investments are made or additional costs are incurred, (for example, through industrial action which damages good relations between management and staff). We address early closure of a project in Chapter 7.

WHEN THINGS GO WRONG: GETTING BACK IN CONTROL

If there is going to be trouble in a project, it tends to rise to the surface during the implementation phase. Sometimes the problems relate directly back to the project design and plan. Perhaps the stakeholder issues are not resolvable, or the decision to proceed in the first place was not a wise one, or the political environment in the organisation is not supportive. No matter what the background to the issues, the project manager is the one whose job it is to sort them out. It is often the ability of the project manager to handle unexpected crises and deviations from the plan that is the determining factor in whether a project is successful or succumbs to the problems that arise during its life.

So when is a project in trouble? The project's monitoring and control activities should provide the project manager with the information required to know its status, and its progress towards objectives at regular intervals. The earlier that signs of trouble are detected the more effectively they can be dealt with. One effective way of avoiding nasty surprises is to have regular reporting both from and to the project team, the steering committee or other stakeholder groups, and the customer or sponsor.

The concrete nature of the project plan (or contract) is intended as a discipline for the sponsor or client as well as for the team. For internal projects, the project plan or the charter can act like a contract, and assist the team to resist unnecessary or harmful 'good ideas' from above.

If problems are emerging, interactions with the project team, the sponsor and stakeholders will contain the warning signs that the project manager needs to assess and respond to. Examples of warning signs that may jeopardise a project include:

- Essential support systems are not working or are significantly behind schedule.
- Senior management is not delivering on promised interventions (such as mandating requirements for staff to participate in training in new systems or procedures).
- The project itself is falling behind schedule to a point where agreed project deliverables will not be met.
- Essential resources (such as provision of IT services) are not forthcoming.
- Stakeholders fail to turn up to important meetings.
- The need for the project outcome is fading because of external changes, or it is losing internal priority.
- The project team is dysfunctional.

- A key person is lost to the project.
- The project objectives are looking unachievable—the outcome will not be sustainable (or profitable) or the service or product will not work well enough.

If signs like these are emerging, decisive action is probably required. Escalating the issue—taking it higher in the organisation—should not be seen by the project manager as a failure, given that many issues arising during the life of the project will be beyond their control. In some cases there will be a need to rethink, and either change the project or close it down (see Chapter 7). In other cases the project manager needs to pull out all stops and 'press on' through a tight spot. Most successful project managers have war stories about projects that succeeded only after great adversity. Sometimes the adversity is a necessary struggle to resolve an unknown or an error in the project design, and in the end it improves the project, though it may also add to the project manager's grey hair.

SUMMARY

- The implementation phase is where the planned project actions are taken and strategies implemented.
- Project mangement is a set of methods but also an art that requires flexibility and persistence. Generic project management skills are important to the success of a project, but familiarity with the content of the project and the culture of the organisation is an advantage.
- Both technical project management skills and people skills are required to be a good project manager.
- Leadership, motivation and teamwork are essential in creating successful project outcomes, in particular team-building skills, running effective meetings and problem-solving skills.
- Projects are powerful enablers of change, and organisational change theorists suggest that participative approaches to change are likely to be more effective and sustainable than top down approaches.
- Managing change is a political process and while some elements of the power structure are overt, many are embedded in the shadow side of the organisation and outside ordinary managerial intervention. Projects can provide an

opportunity to bring important issues into the open and deal constructively with the shadow side.

- Project managers must listen to and understand the dynamics of resistance to change, in particular the forces for and against change, and stakeholder groups.
- Control and monitoring of the progress of project activities (according to the plan) is a key activity in the implementation phase and there are various methods and tools available to do this. The aspects that are monitored during the implementation phase include project scope, schedule, budgets, resources, quality (or performance), risk and contingency.
- The project manager might see warning signs of trouble for the project, and may need to escalate or take these issues higher in the organisation in order for them to be resolved.

7

Closing and evaluation: action, reaction, reflection, action

'Be careful at the end as at the beginning
And there will be no ruined enterprises' (*Lao Tse 1963:125*)

Sooner or later all projects come to an end. For some projects closure comes in an atmosphere of celebration and achievement. For others closure takes place prematurely in an atmosphere of high drama, anger and blame. Projects can even drift along aimlessly until they are quietly killed off behind the scenes when no one is looking. Sometimes projects that have been applauded on completion are found to be wanting when evaluated later. Conversely, projects that appeared to be not so successful on completion can prove their worth at a much later stage. For projects that are trialling a new process or system of work there is always the question of sustainability—will it continue when the project is finally over and there is no project manager in the driving seat?

In this chapter we explore the final stage of the project process, completion and evaluation, and the question of sustainability of project outcomes. First of all we focus on the practical tasks of project completion, followed by a discussion on the dilemmas around the premature closure of projects. We then turn to the evaluation process and ask: Was the project successful? How is that judgment made? and, Will the outcomes last? Finally, we discuss the project report.

WHEN IS A PROJECT FINISHED?

When a project has run its course, the process of completing and closing it (sometimes called 'close-out') is an important final step. Unless the close of a project is actively managed, there can be a tendency for it to drift on, never quite seeming to end. The criteria for project completion are defined (explicitly or implicitly) in the project plan, typically as the finishing of all tasks in the plan, and the achievement of planned outcomes and deliverables. The final tasks could include completing training programs (and the hand-over of training manuals), the installation and commissioning of equipment or the completion of operating manuals (Young 1997).

The key issue is to recognise and move towards a definitive end point, and then tackle the business of completion. The nature of these tasks and their timing will vary, but they fall into three main categories—acceptance and hand-over (the practical completion), evaluation and the final report. If a project is to be killed off, the completion tasks are somewhat different (see later in this chapter).

Acceptance and hand-over

Acceptance and hand-over is the process of practical completion, and includes ensuring that stakeholder expectations have been met, presenting deliverables, winding up the project team and the office, and celebrating success.

Acceptance of the project outcomes or deliverables by the authorised person or group is a key milestone. The team might be handing over an agreed new model of care, a working information system, a new policy and program for staff development, a new method of managing supplies or a new service or program. While all documentation might not yet be finished, practical hand-over of a working or satisfactory outcome should be formalised, even for the smallest and simplest projects. Recognition of the work, and clarity about acceptance, are important for all who have contributed and who will work with the project's outcomes.

A final meeting of the steering committee, or of the team with the project sponsor, is a common method for acceptance and hand-over. Such a meeting can also deal with tying up any loose ends. The project might have brought into focus issues which are outside its scope to resolve and which need to be handed over (for example, participants in community consultations may have identified concerns unrelated to the project which require a response by the agency). There might also be a need to ensure that responsibility for ongoing communication about the project's outcomes is allocated, to cover at least the period while the new process or product is being bedded down.

There may be aspects of the project's deliverables that cannot be wrapped up at the time of completion. A key piece of equipment or software needed for the full operation of a new service might not yet be available, or the industrial implications of a change might have to be sorted out in a different timeframe than was possible in the project. These issues need to be clearly identified, a process for resolving them agreed, and interim arrangements to work around the outstanding issues made.

A debriefing process—that is, an opportunity for people to discuss their experiences and impressions of the project—can be rewarding in itself, and can also provide input to the evaluation and the final report. Members of the steering committee and other key stakeholders, as well as the team, might appreciate opportunities, formal and informal, to debrief.

The team also needs to wind up, even if some members will go on together to work on another project. The project office may need to be closed, and its equipment distributed to the appropriate areas. Individuals sometimes need assistance in the transition back to their old jobs, or in moving on to new ones. Recognition of the transition, and practical assistance, can make it easier. Preparations for this process made in the early stages will pay off at this point.

Finally, there is a need for celebration. A special edition of the agency's newsletter, recording and celebrating the project's outcomes, might be released. A formal hand-over meeting might be followed by a party. The 'go-live' point for a new system delivered by the project can also be the occasion for celebration. The effort and commitment, as well as the achievements, of those who have contributed to a successful outcome need to be recognised. Celebrations of success can be a good way of building or maintaining a positive culture, and can consolidate the pride and satisfaction people feel in their work and their organisation. Parties can also be important when the news is not good, as Case 16 shows.

Case 16: Recognising hand-over in an outsourcing project

The hotel services staff (cleaners, caterers, porters and couriers) of a large health agency had struggled against outsourcing, and had put up an in-house bid (a proposal to keep the service in-house on new terms) which failed. Most of them had been offered jobs by the successful bidder, but there was a lot of sadness and some anger, particularly for the long-serving staff, some of whom had been with the organisation from its beginning, and felt that they had always done a good job.

Care had been taken throughout the project to offer support to the staff, to keep them regularly informed of progress, to facilitate access to independent financial advice, to maximise their opportunities for ongoing employment and to assist those who missed out. The human resources department argued that this approach should be sustained to the end, and that there should be a farewell party for all the staff, whether they were leaving or transferring to the new employer. The CEO agreed, but approached the occasion with dread.

The usual form was to be followed—food and drink, gifts—and a short speech was definitely part of the agenda. With his heart in his mouth, the CEO spoke of the good work and loyalty of the staff, acknowledged that the policy requiring competitive tendering of support services was deeply unpopular, and that the staff had been through a time of uncertainty and anxiety about their futures. He finished by expressing the good wishes of the hospital community. The applause was muted, and the mood sombre, but it was clear that the staff appreciated this proper farewell with the usual courtesies extended. This formal, respectful recognition of the moment of transition may also have contributed to good working relationships under the new contract.

CLOSING DOWN A PROJECT: WHEN PROJECTS FAIL

If a project hasn't succeeded, or is limping along without a clear path to completion, the best course of action may be to abandon or discontinue it. Projects can fail in many ways, from escalation ('just one more extra mile to go') through to seismic shifts in the environment (for example, when a decision to amalgamate two agencies puts more than one developmental project out of business, or at least on a long hold, because amalgamation issues pre-empt them). When the barriers are insurmountable, or when rescue efforts have failed, the only alternative may be to terminate the project, discontinue the work and reassign the people who were working on it.

Closing a project can also be a planned contingency, for example, when the findings in one stage of a project indicate a fatal flaw in its design or feasibility, and the decision not to proceed with further stages is the only option. Some of the more common reasons why projects conclude prematurely are:

- loss of interest and support from management or beneficiaries;
- changing customer requirements, community needs or market conditions;
- indecisiveness, lack of cooperation or support on the part of management or customer or both;
- the project has changed and was no longer able to achieve its original goals;
- chaos and discord from ineffective project management or team conflict; and
- the project outcome itself—that is, the product, did not work, or proved unprofitable. (Lientz and Rea 1998; Kliem et al. 1997).

Terminating a project prior to its planned conclusion is difficult because it usually involves the curtailing of a previously held vision, the breaking up of a 'project family' and perhaps the admission of failure. Termination of a project may simply mean that a project no longer continues in its current form. Meredith and Mantel (2000:540–1) examine the varieties of project termination, terming them extinction, addition, integration and starvation. Extinction means the project is stopped (whether successful or unsuccessful). Addition means that the project is incorporated into ongoing operations as a distinct unit or department in the organisation. Integration is where the project disappears but elements of it are distributed within the organisation, and starvation is where the project still exists but budget cuts mean that no progress is achieved.

Sometimes commitment to a project means that efforts to revive and sustain it continue well beyond the reasonable limits. In a major study of escalation (ever-expanding duration and cost) in IT projects, Keil et al. (2000) surveyed 2500 information systems audit and control professionals. Their results indicate that 30–40 per cent of IT projects escalate, and that once escalation starts ultimate success is much less likely. They also investigated the reasons for persistence with failing projects, and found that 'completion effect', derived from approach avoidance theory, provided the best explanation. That is, projects are more likely to continue when those making decisions believe that they are so close to completion that persistence is justified regardless of additional cost. The implication is that once an IT project begins seriously to fail, it is probably best to let it go.

In health and community services, it may be that passion as well as completion effect influence poor decision making when projects are in trouble. We have already highlighted the issue of commitment to a worthy goal in the absence of feasible means, and the problem of conflicting goals and incentives. Avoidance of terminating can mean that projects are left to stagnate—neither progressing towards their initial goals and objectives nor moving towards closure.

While the process of termination is never easy, it should be done quickly to minimise further waste of resources and disruption to the organisation. Terminating a project is not likely to be the sole decision of any one person, but rather the result of a series of discussions where the project, and its progress, are evaluated unfavourably.

One exit method for a project that is limping to a dead end is simply to declare it finished—adopt a modified goal and cut the losses, with as much dignity as possible. Recommendations for follow-up activity might be made, and evaluation might enable the lessons to be learnt from the experience. The team should be thanked for their efforts and resettled, with perhaps an opportunity for the drowning of sorrows.

When the failure is irrefutable, it is often a good idea to develop and articulate a clear statement of reasons, and proactively communicate this message to all concerned, without delay and as consistently as possible. This tactic will not stop rumours, but it will at least ensure that they are not circulated in a vacuum. The rights and interests of the staff involved need to be protected, without delay.

169

WHAT IS PROJECT SUCCESS?

The operational definition of project success, like the project itself, is unique. While the generic 'iron triangle' of cost, time and specifications is a useful reference point, real projects have more flavour and texture, as well as outcomes which go beyond the project deliverables (and even their quality and efficacy). As Lientz and Rea suggest, 'Project success is a vague term. A project could be a physical failure, but a political success ... success depends on the perspective from which the project is viewed' (1998:315).

Lientz and Rea (1998) propose these criteria for judging success:

- Is the end product (or project outcome) being used?
- How well did the project manager and project team perform?

And we would add the following:

- How effective or sustainable was the change process?
- Were all the project objectives met?
- Was the impact (both long and short term) on patients/clients or the organisation positive?

Many of our respondents, when asked about project failures or elements of a project that did not meet goals, took a holistic view of the project in its context and judged success broadly, on the basis of more than the specific project objectives. The respondents were equally concerned about things like the project's impact on the organisation as a whole, organisational learning, communication and skill development, retention of valuable staff, and cultural and practice change.

Several respondents were reluctant to admit that a project had failed but rather suggested that while some aspects of the project could be improved upon, or 'done differently next time', the overall project experience was beneficial for the organisation. This perception of the value of even unsuccessful projects perhaps arose partly from a natural reluctance to focus on failure. Respondents also seemed to be relying on a philosophy (in relation to project management and continuous quality improvement) whereby project outcomes were viewed both as learning opportunities and as part of a cumulative experience of change and innovation across the whole organisation.

Whatever the complexities of defining success for each project, it is important that success is acknowledged. It is also important that the criteria by which the project's outcomes will be judged are determined, preferably in the evaluation section of the project plan, and form the basis for the evaluation.

WHY DO EVALUATION?

The majority of the project management literature advocates formal review and evaluation of projects—often called a 'post-implementation review'. Evaluation involves making judgments about something against a set of agreed criteria (Wilson and Wright 1993:2). An evaluation not only provides some answers to the question 'Did we do what we set out to do?' but enables the lessons of the project, both good and bad, to be learned and applied to future projects and programs, and provides an opportunity to reflect on outcomes, processes, organisation and methods. Evaluation can assist in completing a change process by consolidating both the evidence for the change and a common understanding of what it means. Evaluation can be a powerful method of building cumulative knowledge for later projects.

'Insider evaluation' is carried out by the project team themselves with input from the key stakeholders. For the people involved, participation in evaluation assists in the process of finishing and moving on. Insider evaluation has the benefit of the participants' intimate knowledge and understanding of the project. It can encourage the development of critical reflection skills and assist in embedding these skills within the organisation itself. However, insider evaluation might be viewed as biased and therefore invalid or of less value than evaluation by others. And it might be less rigorous, since participants often want their project to look good and will dwell more on the positives, perhaps downplaying the negatives (Wilson and Wright 1993:5).

Evaluation is often carried out by 'outsiders', perhaps a group of skilled specialists in a particular methodology or approach (for example, economic evaluation). Outsider evaluation is often seen as more credible but it is also more costly and is likely to be used only for larger projects.

It is important to consider who the evaluation is for—in other words, who are the key stakeholders? As well as the organisation and the project team, potential interested parties might include the providers of funds, other agencies, service users, industry associations and government departments.

As we stressed in Chapter 5, evaluation should be built into every project at the planning stage. In reality, however, resistance to undertaking a formal project evaluation is common, and many of the organisations interviewed for our research indicated that formalised project evaluations were mostly not done. There are several reasons for this. Project reviews without specific objectives can turn into witch-hunts, and looking transparently at things that went wrong or need improvement is very confronting. The pressure to focus on the next goal or task undoubtedly also contributes.

Another common issue in health and community services is the underlying approach to evaluation of programs and services in general. The health sector in particular is a science-based industry, with traditional approaches to research and evaluation based on the controlled experiment. This involves holding most elements constant while testing one element of interest (Wilson and Wright 1993:xii). There was a perceived tendency in our study (particularly in health care agencies) to regard anything less than gold-standard evaluation as not worth doing. One senior manager referred to the preference for rigorous methods like the randomised controlled trial as a barrier against evaluating at all.

Yet evaluation is critical. When the project has a direct impact on patient or client care, evaluation should be mandatory, to assess the impact and ensure that there are no adverse effects on standards or access for the target population. Even if the outcome is not direct, a good evaluation process can be a valuable aid to organisational learning and future practice.

Some writers have criticised the use of traditional 'scientific' approaches to evaluation in health and community services, arguing that they are not appropriate for projects influenced by complex social and political networks and relationships (Patton 1990; Wadsworth 1990). They argue that naturalistic and interpretative methodologies are more valuable. Often described as qualitative research or evaluation, the methods include unstructured and semi-structured interviews with key players, direct and indirect observation, focus groups and case studies.

In reality a range of methods and data collection techniques can be employed. This is likely to include 'hard' or quantitative data such as occupational health and safety or workforce statistics, and data on performance as well as the softer, more qualitative approaches. As Patton (1990:9) argues: 'There are no rigid rules that can be provided for making data collection and methods decisions in evaluation. The art of evaluation involves creating a design and gathering information that is appropriate for a specific situation and a particular policy-making context.' The important point is that the project evaluation design is included as part of the project planning phase, so that the right information can be collected in the right way for that project as part of its implementation.

A FRAMEWORK FOR PROJECT EVALUATION

Project evaluation basically asks, 'Did we do what we set out to do?' We have already said that there is not one way of doing it, but there are three recognised categories of evaluation based on goals, objectives and strategies (Hawe et al. 1990:43–4):

- *Process evaluation* measures the effectiveness of the strategies and methods used in the project, and the skill of their execution. In a health promotion project it will probably include the views of the participants as to their satisfaction with the intervention.
- *Impact evaluation* measures achievement of the program objectives and sub-objectives. It focuses on the short-term impact and is usually related to the project's objectives but can also include unforeseen and unanticipated events whether beneficial or detrimental.
- *Outcome evaluation* measures achievement of the long-term project goals.

As Hawe et al. (1990:103) point out, impact and outcome evaluation both assess the effects of the completed intervention, but over different time periods. Impact evaluation is an assessment of the immediate effects whereas outcome evaluation looks at the later or longer-term effects, and usually relates to the original goal.

In reality, outcome evaluation is hardly ever possible in the timeframes that apply to projects. This means that the hard evidence for the effectiveness of interventions in the system of service delivery is not often produced. One senior public servant we interviewed noted this problem: 'What we are trying to do is promote the uptake of innovation, promote change, promote the identification of better ways of doing things and then promote the uptake of these better things. And there is a life cycle there that is longer than the phase of the program. So in the end can you reliably evaluate the program's effectiveness in an evaluation that is contemporaneous with the program? I suspect not. Because you can't at the time pick up how well it is going to be sustained and you certainly can't pick up its system impact, the systemic effect.'

A management consultant was pragmatic on this question: 'We evaluate internally, with the team—Is the client happy, is it in budget and on time? What did we learn? Clients generally specify in great detail how they'll evaluate the tender bids, but have not much to say about how they evaluate project outcomes.' A health service CEO was blunt: 'It is mostly not done.'

Impact evaluation can be a simple procedure. As the director of a women's health service put it: 'Having a new system in place that works is the best evaluation. The criterion is "Does it work?" and the answer we need is "Yes".' Surrogate indicators can also make the impact of complex changes measurable. In talking about a large project which introduced a new model of care, the project leader noted: 'Sick leave was a very good indicator that we were actually getting some attitudinal change. It halved within the first six months of the project and it stayed down, compared with the rest of the organisation, for the rest of the project and is now going down again a bit more.'

Process evaluation might often be the most feasible. It is often relatively straightforward to write standards or criteria for assessing the processes of a project as it unfolds. Giving people real time feedback on what is happening can also enhance the project's chances of success. A senior project manager commented: 'You need to actually give people real-time feedback, not three-months-late feedback. One of the mistakes we made is that we only evaluated process at the six months' point. The feedback took three months to get and by that time most people had moved on and the opportunity for assessing it was long gone. I don't think it needs to be complex and I don't think there is any magic formula, it really depends on what you are trying to do. It is better to give them half information on time than the full information in months.'

Case 17: Evaluation in the community setting

A community health service had a request from a local GP concerning the needs of an increasing number of Afghani women attending her surgery. She felt that their needs were largely social and emotional rather than medical and asked 'Could you do something for them?' The agency met with the women's unofficial interpreter, and after much discussion set up a project to establish an Afghani Women's Health Program in the area. The project had three major objectives: first, to identify the health needs of Afghani women, second to develop strategies to meet those needs, and third to raise awareness among other service providers in the area.

Discussion groups were held, resources were collected, and an Afghani Women's Health Forum was conducted, with invited speakers addressing important cultural and health issues. Other activities followed. Service providers in the area took part, and were successfully engaged in broader responses to the needs of the group.

The project was evaluated in a number of ways. As the project leader said: 'We first of all asked the question "Did we do what we set out to do—that is, did we establish the program?" The answer to that question was clearly, "Yes". Second, we collected data on the numbers of women and service providers attending all the activities, and we collected demographic data about the range of women attending —age, education, etc. Third, we asked for feedback from all participants in our activities through both participant feedback sheets and group discussion. Finally, we involved the Afghani women in decision making about future activities, thus reflecting on what we had done and identifying what worked and what didn't. In this way we carried out both impact and process evaluation—we just did what seemed logical.'

An outcome evaluation of the project—that is, of its contribution to the better health of the women involved —was not possible, because the timeframe and the complexity of measuring health outcomes were beyond its scope. However, the project had both unforeseen and longer-term impacts. For example, the women identified a whole range of issues as important to their health, such as housing, immigration, work and education, which went well beyond the issues the agency had initially considered. The women also organised among themselves and became very involved in local housing issues. One woman went on to open her own restaurant, actively supported by the others.

There was also an impact on service providers, who were made aware of the group's needs and of the need to change some of their practice if they were to be able to service the needs of such a group. This realisation led to a series of cultural awareness projects in some of the mainstream agencies.

But there was another way the staff knew that the project had been a success. 'When they came to hold their meetings they filled the place up with laughter, colour, food and good energy. That good energy lifted the spirits of everyone else in the place—hard to explain in evaluation terms but easy to see and feel in practice.'

THE FINAL REPORT

The final report is an important element in closing a project and summing it up, either as part of acceptance and hand-over, or at the post-implementation review stage. Usually written by the project manager, the final report details the overall project at the point of completion and is useful as:

- a good historical record of the project and what it achieved;
- an opportunity for reflection on the project as a whole;
- a comparison of the project at completion with the plan;
- a way of informing stakeholders of the status of any outstanding issues;
- a record of recommendations for future projects and strategies for sustaining the outcomes of this project; and
- a summary of what went right and what went wrong, to promote learning for subsequent projects.

A good final report is structured so that the reader can get a clear overview quickly, can easily find particular information of interest, and doesn't get lost in the detail. While the size and structure of the report will depend on the nature of the project, the sections or headings shown in Figure 13 might provide a useful starting point:

The project report should not be structured as a chronological record of the project process (the 'what I did on my holidays' approach). Rather it should be logically structured in the way that best meets the knowledge and decision-making needs of the readers, avoids repetition, enables the reader to assess the quality and import of the information and data, and hopefully persuades them to agree with the team's conclusions and recommendations.

The project report is usually more than a record of what happened in the project. If the report needs to convince decision makers to adopt a proposed change or sustain a project outcome, the logic of its structure should be designed to lead the reader to agree with its proposals. One model is the 'problem/solution' model: 'the problem is "x"; the possible ways of addressing it are "a, b and c"; we've done a lot of work to determine that "b" is the best method of solving the problem; and the agency should do "y" to ensure this outcome'.

The 'opportunity knocks' model is similar, but applies when the task is to take advantage of an opportunity. The logic is developed along the lines of: 'we are currently doing "x" to achieve "y"; new information/technology/policy/funding provides the opportunity to do "x" better/at higher volume/at lower cost/differently, or achieve something greater through doing something other than "x"; and therefore the agency should do "z" to secure this advantage'.

If the report is needed to meet the accountability requirements of a funding body (including corporate head office), the author needs to be aware of what their expectations are, and strive to meet them.

A well-written report is a lot more convincing than one that leaves the reader to disentangle spelling errors, poor grammar and unclear meaning. Writing the contents page first is one way to focus on clear, logical structuring. Some writers find it useful to outline the report first using dot points, others prefer to draft whole sections or paragraphs and move them around later if necessary. For most people, there is no real substitute for drafting, reading (and preferably getting others to read) and redrafting, and modern word processing packages make this process much easier.

Figure 13: Final report template

Cover

Organisational logo

Name of project

Date of report or submission

Contents page

Executive summary

- Maximum 2–3 pages giving an overview of project goals, methods, outcomes, achievements and any recommendations or future implications

Report sections

- Introduction — project background and purpose; the project 'story'
- Project goals and methods — including resourcing, sponsor, team, project organisation, committee, etc.
- Outcomes and key achievements — using the evaluation outcomes
- Issues — arising from the project but not resolved by it
- Sustaining the outcomes — recommendations and action required
- Summary of key project data and performance indicators — if not included in the relevant sections above

References

Appendices

- Key project documents as appendices

The project report may need to conform to a house style for documents. The sources of ideas and assertions in the report should be acknowledged, and this is becoming more important as agencies pursue the goals of evidence-based practice and evidence-based decision making. There are many acceptable referencing styles, and the agency may have a preferred style. The most important thing is to use it consistently, including for information and documents found on the internet.

If there is a wealth of important detail, it should be organised into attachments so that this data is available for those who need it (perhaps in the form of a separate volume with limited circulation). If the report has a practical use after the life of the project, it may be worthwhile to budget for a professional editor—readability can be significantly improved at a fairly modest cost.

Tips for effective presentations

Some organisations require simpler documentation, perhaps little more than a set of presentation slides. In any organisation, a clear, concise presentation on overhead projector or data projector is an effective way of communicating the project's outcomes and implications, and is a valuable adjunct to the written report. It can be worthwhile doing this well, as a good presentation can be used repeatedly to ensure that a clear, consistent message about the project is communicated to all those affected or interested in its outcomes. These are some tips for effective presentations:

- Show an outline slide right after the title slide. It gives the overall structure of the presentation and helps the audience know where you're taking them.
- 'Tell them what you're going to tell them, tell them, then tell them what you've told them' is an old adage for getting your message across. That is, give an outline, give your message, then sum up.
- The slides/overheads are like a skeleton—they're the structure of your presentation. All your major points should be summarised on the slides, and their relationships should be clear (for example, subpoints, correct order, etc.). They help the audience to

follow your logic and know where you are heading. They also help the presenter to 'step through' the presentation.

■ Put a minimum of words on each slide. Summarise your points, don't include the full text. Each slide should have a maximum of about six lines of text, or a diagram or picture. Do not read your slides word for word, unless there's an especially good quote, or a punch line.

■ The rule of thumb is one slide per minute. If you've got 15 minutes to present, you should have about 15 slides.

■ The bigger the better for text size—no text should be less than 20 point size, otherwise it's not readable.

■ On a data projector, dark backgrounds and light print seem to work best. The opposite holds true for old-fashioned overheads. Whichever way you go, have a strong contrast between the background and the text—black on red, for example, is hard to read.

■ Face the audience and make eye contact. It is very tempting to focus on the overheads—by turning around and looking at the wall—and then the audience sees the back of your head. When you need to check your slides, look either at the computer screen, or at the overhead on the projector—then you only need to look down rather than turn your back.

■ Find a place to stand so that the audience can see both you and the screen.

■ Try to relax and focus on communicating with the audience—rely on good preparation to support you while you get your message across.

Formal hand-over of the final report should also be considered. For some projects it is useful to produce a short summary document for general communication of outcomes within the organisation and among its stakeholders. Distribution of such a document also brings an opportunity to thank those who participated in workshops, interviews or consultations, and demonstrates that their input was valued.

Sustaining Project Outcomes

Sustaining the project outcomes can be difficult when the project team disperses and funding is exhausted. In an environment of scarce resources it is tempting to pursue one's dreams for better or bigger services using small dollops of project funding in order to make a start on what may turn out to be a long journey, requiring ongoing support and resources.

The question of sustainability should be addressed at the concept stage, and dispassionate decisions are needed at that point. While there are good reasons for tilting at windmills very occasionally, to do so routinely is to dissipate energy, reputation, capacity and support. Our research indicates that the tendency to take on impossible or improbable challenges is a real problem for some organisations in the sector.

There are many aspects of sustainability that the project itself cannot influence—emerging budget problems, for example. One of the important sustainability variables where the project can make a difference seems to be the extent of engagement of those who will be responsible for ongoing operations. If members of the future operational team are involved in the project concept, design, planning and implementation, they are more likely to be enthusiastic implementers of the outcomes.

Where the project is someone else's good idea, or is operated in a way which excludes or frustrates the receiving team, sustainability is more likely to be a rocky road. This has implications for the way in which central project units conduct their work, and emphasises again the importance of skilled engagement with stakeholders and recognition of their legitimate interests in the detailed working arrangements of the project.

We have also discussed earlier the use of projects as seduction—persuading others to act by showing how a good idea can work in practice. If such a project succeeds, its existence changes the balance of probabilities (and increases the costs of refusing funding) when ongoing resources are being divided up. Case 18 illustrates the point.

Case 18: Sustaining the unsustainable

An emergency response service in a teaching hospital was funded as a project on the theory that if it worked, it would save the hospital costs (by preventing admissions) and would therefore be self-sustaining. The project was evaluated by a major consulting firm, which found that the funding hypothesis was correct in the sense that enough admissions were avoided to cover the direct costs of providing the service. They also found that the money was not in fact available for transfer to pay for the service, because the number of admissions to the hospital was not reduced—other patients took the place of those assisted by the service.

However, the service was very popular with patients (who were able to go home with support) and with staff (who were able to move more patients through the emergency department in a timely manner). It had also been given positive coverage in the local media and was written up in an academic journal. Some of the patients became aware that the funding base was fragile and lobbied for its continuation. The end result was that the service was sustained on repeated rounds of temporary funding for at least five years.

A successful project can also work to improve the chances of a supportive policy decision being made. It is easier for governments or health authorities to make policy supporting innovative services, or interventions in social problems, if they can point to the results of a successful trial. The success of needle exchange programs in reducing the rate of HIV infection in intravenous drug users is an example of this—the idea of handing out equipment for use in an illegal activity is otherwise hard to justify.

While there are many excellent examples of this strategy—'show it can work and then get the money (or the policy change)'—embarking on this course is a significant risk. It should be done knowingly, for very good reasons, and as an exception not the rule.

SUMMARY

- Project closure is an important step in the project life cycle and needs to be actively managed. This phase includes acceptance and hand-over of the project outcomes and deliver-ables to the authorised person or group.

■ Activities in project closure include a final meeting and the submission of a final report. Recognising and celebrating the efforts and achievements of those involved in the project, and planning for life after the project, are important.

■ Projects can fail for a variety of reasons, and may require early termination. While this can be difficult, there are situations where premature closure is the best available course of action.

■ Evaluation of projects in the health and community services sector is important, but need not be elaborate. There are a range of methods and data collection techniques for both process and outcome evaluation.

■ Sustaining the outcomes of a project can be difficult, but it is more likely to occur where members of the future oper-ational team are involved in the project concept, design, planning and implementation, and where they can become change champions.

Conclusion
Organisational learning
and keeping on track

'It is not only knowledge we are concerned with but all the processes of learning, imagination, creation, performance.' (*Williams 1980:29*)

We conclude with some thoughts about how the learnings and capabilities developed through good projects and good project management are embedded in organisations. We also offer some thoughts about the future development of project management in the sector.

Throughout this book we have emphasised the need for genuine organisational commitment to the project, for a well-developed and feasible project plan, for adequate resources and a high-performing project team. We found that in practice project management in a complex industry is not just a set of competencies that can be taught from a manual but requires flexibility, understanding and good judgment.

Good judgment is not something that can be learnt from a textbook; good judgment comes from experience and a willingness to reflect and learn from that experience. As Legge and Stanton (2002) point out, 'Where managers have real choices they cannot *know* the right answer; they have to rely on their judgment (and this means taking risks).'

However, taking risks can be tempered through reflection on practice, and choosing between different strategies involves recognition of similar experiences—what worked and what did not. The more we reflect and learn from our personal practice the greater chance we have of making improved decisions when faced with complex situations.

ORGANISATIONAL LEARNING

Exactly the same principle applies to teams, departments and organisations. 'Most companies are investing heavily in innovative project work but investing nothing in evaluating and learning from it' (Disterer 2002:513). This is not only a waste in time and resources but it is also a missed opportunity for organisational development. Many organisations are capable of what Agryris (1992) describes as single-loop learning—that is, detecting and fixing errors and problems within the existing system. However, they are not always so good at double-loop learning, which challenges the underlying system and its assumptions, and asks 'Why do we do this in this way? Is there a better way?' The concept of organisational learning has something to offer here.

Organisational learning is an intuitively appealing but slightly tricky concept. It uses the learning process of individuals as a metaphor for the way organisations acquire, store and use information and experience. It is intuitively appealing because most people who have worked in organisations have experienced the benefits of the special embedded knowledge and skills which the organisation itself, as opposed to the sum of its members, seems to hold. For example, Family Planning Associations seem to 'know' how to work with very young clients in the complex area of sexuality and contraception without getting into problems with consent. Management in complex situations calls for organisations that have such embedded collective knowledge.

Senge (1992) constructs the elements of organisational learning in terms of five disciplines: personal mastery, mental models, shared vision, team learning and (the fifth discipline) systems thinking. Organisational learning can be understood at different levels. At the level of the individual practitioner it may mean simply being able to keep up with current research and practice in his or her field. The chances of success are enhanced if management can ensure that the conditions are right for the staff of the organisation to keep learning at this individual level (Legge and Stanton 2002).

At the level of systems and procedures, organisational learning can be thought about in terms of the idea of self-organising reform. Self-directed teams are the foundation of a learning organisation and problem solving is a fundamental approach. In a learning organisation teams, networks and alliances whose work is linked in various ways across the organisation think collectively about better ways of working. They innovate, evaluate and remodel, and they orient their own reforms within a wider view of where they fit into the organisation's purposes and values, and current movements in the broader environment (Legge and Stanton 2002).

But organisational learning is tricky because organisations do not have brains, and too literal use of individual learning as a metaphor can be misleading. For example, organisational knowledge needs different methods of sharing, management, renewal and encoding from the knowledge of individuals.

So how does all this relate to project management? Projects are seen as 'learning intensive organisational forms' (Disterer 2002:512) but Disterer and others (e.g. Weiser and Morrison 1998) note that the boundaries between projects and the ongoing functions of the organisation can act as barriers against organisational learning from projects. This reality is seen, for example, in the fact that evaluation is rarely about improving project management practices, and that project files are stored without reference to ease of future use. Indeed, some of the lessons from project experiences are actively rejected by organisations—for example, when their implications cause discomfort because they do not fit with the espoused culture and values. Argyris (1992) describes this behaviour in terms of organisational defence mechanisms; perhaps there are 'undiscussables'—certain issues that cannot be addressed for reasons everyone has forgotten. The organisation might also act out a number of defensive routines, for example, organising meetings that identify issues but never resolve them, instead passing them on to a proliferation of other meetings and committees (Delahaye 2000:52).

In human services, where professional and organisational knowledge are so vital to the core functions of organisations, it is important for these barriers to be addressed. The approach now called 'knowledge management' provides some good insights into how this might be done. Knowledge management recognises that an organisation's knowledge is a major asset, and aims to exploit intellectual capital in an organisation through leveraging and reusing all information and knowledge, and encouraging organisational learning. It is defined as all activities to understand, focus on and manage systematic, explicit and deliberate knowledge-building, renewal and application (Wiig 1997, cited in Disterer 2002).

Because projects are specifically designed to be temporary efforts, the knowledge gained typically disperses with the team. There are some fairly simple steps that can be taken to counteract this tendency:

- An internal 'yellow pages' could be started, listing project staff in categories of their project assignments and expertise (Hansen et al. 1999).
- In larger organisations with project support units, the role of collecting knowledge from projects could be centralised.
- The project team could generate a short bulletin summarising the major learnings from the project to be stored on the organisation's intranet or in its library.
- Project team mentor roles could be fostered among experienced project managers.

Capturing the lessons and contributions to organisational knowledge arising from projects is an outstanding challenge for many organisations.

NOT ANOTHER MANAGEMENT FAD: KEEPING PROJECT MANAGEMENT ON TRACK

As we were finishing writing, we heard a worrying story from a senior project manager in a Department of Health. In Case 19 she describes the devastation of project 'scope creep' imposed from above.

Case 19: Project 'scope creep': risks from above

We were presenting a progress report to five members of the Department's executive on a project which had been commissioned by the full executive with very clearly specified deliverables and timelines, and it was going pretty well. It was a Friday afternoon and I thought we might end the week on a high note. We hadn't got very far into the presentation when one of the directors had a good idea—off the top of his head—which had the effect of significantly broadening the scope of the project. Maybe the planets were badly aligned, but the others joined in, so I attempted to point out the implications and gently remind them about the importance of sticking to the project goals and timeframe. I lost, and we were told, 'Well, it's not worth doing the thing if you're not going to do it as well as possible.' The Department does have a project management protocol, and it is very clear that this sort of intervention is not supposed to happen, or at least, not without consequences. But I know for certain that I can't now prepare a variation and ask for approval without being seen as an uncooperative spoiler. We'll muddle through, I suppose, but we all went back to the office and started polishing our résumés. It was really exasperating to be so seriously highjacked by the very people who'd approved the project and insisted on tight timelines.

This experience is a sobering example of the way in which any management method or tool can be misinterpreted or misused. The last 20 years have seen a steady stream of new management methods sweep industry generally, and usually spread to human services—total quality management, business process re-engineering, organisational restructuring and many more. Some authors see these as simply repackaging of useful management practices and at worst expensive distractions from the business of solving organisational problems (Egan 1994:xiv).

We have lived through many of these management fads, and have come to the conclusion that there is a common story of reduction. An organisation, assisted perhaps by consultants or academics, faces up to a serious problem and works to solve it. In various ways they refocus the organisation on its purpose, its real reason for existing, while also developing some kind of break-through in thinking or method. Word spreads, perhaps through the efforts of consultants and academics, or perhaps mandated by corporate head offices or government departments, and others take up the method. Sooner rather than later, other organisations start using the method without having gone through the rethinking process, looking only for a quick fix to a problem, or to conform to a directive, or not to be left behind. The success achieved by the inventors and early adopters is not sustained, and after a while the method is criticised for failing to deliver on its promise.

The apparent vulnerability of management to faddism can be seen as a symptom of a deeper problem—the devaluing of well-established management knowledge and corruption of the professional practice of management (Hilmer and Donaldson 1996). Hilmer and Donaldson argue that there is no substitute for hard, clear thinking and sustained effort, 'the disciplined application of fundamental concepts guided by values and reasoned analysis' (1996:xiv).

Will project management go this way? Will we see, for example, a new round of prescriptions and the reduction of project management to a set of hurdles that have to leapt through before funding can be approved? The prescribing of PRINCE2 by the government in the UK (Roberts and Ludvigsen, 1998) is a worrying step in this direction.

THE LAST WORD

We hope that this book will contribute in a small way to averting that potential future, and supporting instead the realisation of three key enhancements arising from project management methods. First, we hope to see more professional and managerial staff in human service organisations add the project approach to their repertoire of problem-solving methods, particularly where significant changes in ways of delivering or supporting their core services are needed. Awareness of practical issues like the need for planning and the usefulness of tools like process-mapping and risk management might then be widely disseminated and become part of usual practice.

Second, more senior managers and professional leaders might accept the discipline of project management in their own approaches to managing change and development. This would mean greater clarity and openness about goals and methods, willingness to support skill development, better understanding that 'the devil is in the detail', and greater respect for the real work of project teams.

Finally, we hope that organisations will be better able to achieve their goals and meet the needs of their stakeholders because they have developed effective ways of getting their good ideas to work.

References

Alsene, E. (1998). 'Internal changes and project management structures within enterprises', *International Journal of Project Management* 17(6): 367–76

Argyris, C. (1992). *On Organizational Learning*, Blackwell, Cambridge, Mass.

Ayas, K. (1996). 'Professional project management: A shift towards learning and a knowledge creating structure', *International Journal of Project Management* 14(3): 131–6

Belassi, W. and Tukel, O. (1996). 'A new framework for determining critical success/failure factors in projects', *International Journal of Project Management* 14(3): 141–51

Bennett, C., Coffey, S., McDonald, B. and McNeal, B. (2001). Planning and Evaluating Collaborative Research and Extension, *www.reeusda.gov/pas/resources/integrative*

Brody, R. (2000). *Effectively Managing Human Service Organisations,* 2nd edn, Sage Publications, Thousand Oaks, CA (see Chapter 15, Team Building and Coalition Building, pp. 287–305)

Carter, R. and Harris, A. (1999). 'Evaluation of health services' in G. Mooney and R. Scotton (eds), *Economics and Australian Health Policy,* Allen & Unwin, Sydney

Case, R. (1998). 'The structure of high-performing project management organisations', *Drug Information Journal* 32: 577–607

Central Computer and Telecommunications Agency (CCTA) (1997). *PRINCE 2: An Outline*, Norwich, UK

Chapman, P. and Davey, P. (1997). 'Working "with" communities, not "on" them: A changing focus for local government health planning in Queensland', *Australian Journal of Primary Health Interchange* 3(1): 82–91

Chittenden, R.A. (1997). 'Caltrans' quest for "true project management" in government bureaucracy', in J. Meredith and S. Mantel (2000). *Project Management: A managerial approach,* 4th edn, J. Wiley & Sons, New York, pp. 159–60

Commonwealth of Australia (2000). *Improving Health Services Through Consumer Participation: A resource guide for organisations,* National Resource Centre for Consumer Participation in Health, Melbourne, *http://www.participateinhealth.org.au/clearinghouse/*

De Fillipi, R.J. (2001). 'Introduction: Project-based learning reflective practices and learning outcomes', *Management Learning* 32(1): 5–10 (Special Issue)

Delahaye, B. (2000). *Human Resource Development: Principles and practice,* Wiley & Sons, Brisbane

Department of Health and Ageing (2002). *Supporting Innovation in Patient Care: NDHP,* Canberra, Commonwealth of Australia

Department of Industry, Science and Resources (2000). Shaping Australia's Future Innovations—Framework Paper, Commonwealth of Australia, Canberra

DeSimone, R., Werner, J. and Harris, D. (2002). *Human Resource Development,* 3rd edn, Harcourt Brace, Fort Worth

Disterer, G. (2002). 'Management of project knowledge and experiences', *Journal of Knowledge Management,* 6(5): 512–20

Dobson, M. (1996). *Practical Project Management: The secrets of managing any project on time and on budget,* Skillpath Publications, Mission, Kansas

Drummond, M.F., O'Brien, B.J., Stoddart, G.L. and Torrance, G.W. (1997). *Methods for the Economic Evaluation of Health Care Programmes,* Oxford University Press

Dunford, R. (1992). *Organisational Behaviour: An organisational analysis perspective,* Addison-Wesley, Sydney

Dunphy, D. and Stace, D. (1990). *Under New Management: Australian organisations in transition,* McGraw-Hill, Sydney

Dwyer, J. and Leggat, S. (2002). 'Innovation in Australian hospitals', *Australian Health Review* 25(5): 19–31

Egan, G. (1994). *Working the Shadow Side: A guide to positive behind the scenes management,* Jossey Bass, San Francisco

Gold, M.R., Siegal, J.E., Russell, L.B., Weinstein, M.C. (eds) (1996). *Cost Effectiveness in Health and Medicine (Report of the Washington Panel on Cost Effectiveness in Health and Medicine),* Oxford University Press, New York

Halligan, A. and Donaldson, L. (2001). 'Implementing clinical governance: Turning vision into reality', *British Medical Journal* 9 June, 322(7299): 1413

Hart, C. (1998). *Doing a Literature Review: Releasing the social science research imagination,* Sage Publications, London

Hawe, P., Degeling, D. and Hall, J. (1990). *Evaluating Health Promotion,* MacLennan & Petty, Sydney

Hayes, H.B. (2002). 'Using earned-value analysis for better project management', *Biopharm* March 2002, pp. 58–60

Haynes, M. (1994). *Project Management: From idea to implementation*, Crisp Publications, UK

Healy, P. (1997). *Project Management: Getting the job done on time and on budget*, Butterworth Heinemann, Melbourne

Hilmer, F.G. and Donaldson, L. (1996). *Management Redeemed: Debunking the fads that undermine corporate performance*, The Free Press, Sydney.

Hood, C. (1991). 'A public management for all seasons?', *Public Administration* 69(1): 3–19

Jang, Y. and Lee, J. (1998). 'Factors influencing the success of management consulting projects', *International Journal of Project Management* 16(2): 67–72

Kahn, E.F. (1982). 'Critical themes in the study of change', in P.S. Goodman and associates (eds), *Change in Organisations*, Jossey Bass, San Francisco, pp. 409–29

Keil, M., Mann, J. and Rai, A. (2000). 'Why software projects escalate: an empirical analysis and test of four theoretical models', *MIS Quarterly*, 24(4): 631–64

Kerzner, H. (1998). *In Search of Excellence in Project Management: Successful practices in high performance organisations,* Van Nostrand Reinhold, New York

Kliem, R., Ludin, I. and Robertson, K. (1997). *Project Management Methodology: A practical guide for the next millennium*, Marcel Dekker Inc., New York

Kotter, J. and Schlesinger, L. (1979). 'Choosing strategies for change', *Harvard Business Review* March–April, pp. 106–14

Kumar, R. (1996). *Research Methodology*, Longman, Melbourne

Lao Tse (1963). *Ta Te Ching*, Penguin, London

Leggat, S. and Dwyer, J. (2003). 'Factors supporting high performance in health care organisations: A review of the literature', *National Institute of Clinical Studies, http://www.nicsl.com.au/resources_reports.asp?cat=27&navPage=2*

Legge, D. and Stanton, P. (2002). 'Learning management (and managing your own learning)', pp. 1–24 in M. Harris, *Managing Health Services: Concepts and practice*, MacLennan & Petty, Sydney

Lewin, K. (1958). 'Group decisions and social change', in E. Maccoby (ed), *Readings in Social Psychology*, Holt, Rinehart & Winston, New York

Lientz, B. and Rea, K. (1998). *Project Management for the 21st Century*, 2nd edn, Academic Press, San Diego

Limerick, D. and Cunnington, B. (1993). *Managing the New Organization: A blueprint for networks and alliances*, Jossey Bass, San Franscisco

Lock, D. (2001). *The Essentials of Project Management*, 2nd edn, Gower Publishing Limited, Hampshire, UK

Martin, V. and Henderson, E. (2001). *Managing in Health and Social Care*, Routledge, London

Maylor, H. (1996). *Project Management*, Pitman Publishing, London

McElroy, W. (1996). 'Implementing strategic change through projects', *International Journal of Project Management* 14(6): 325–9

Meredith, J. and Mantel, S. (2000). *Project Management: A managerial approach*, 4th edn, J. Wiley & Sons Inc., New York

Mintzberg, H. (1991). 'Ideology and the missionary organisation', in H. Mintzberg and B. Quinn, *The Strategy Process: Concepts, contexts, cases*, Prentice-Hall, Englewood Cliffs, New Jersey, pp. 352–8

Mintzberg, H. and Quinn, M. (1991). *The Strategy Process: Concepts, contexts, cases*, Prentice-Hall, Englewood Cliffs, New Jersey

Muir Gray, J.A. (1997). *Evidence-based Healthcare: How to make health policy and management decisions*, Churchill Livingstone, Edinburgh

Nadler, D. and Tushman, M. (1997). 'Implementing new designs: managing organizational change', in M. Tushman and P. Anderson (eds), *Managing Strategic Innovation and Change: A collection of readings*, Oxford University Press, New York

NHS (National Health Strategy) (1993). *Pathways to Better Health*, Canberra: NHS

O'Kelly, S.W. and Maxwell, R. (2001). 'Implementing clinical governance. Medical training should include project management', *British Medical Journal* 323(7315): 753

Partington, D. (1996). 'The project management of organizational change', *International Journal of Project Management* 14(1): 13–21

Patton, M.Q. (1990). *Qualitative Evaluation and Research Methods*, Sage Publications, Thousand Oaks, CA

Perce, K.H. (1998). 'Project management skills', *Australian Association of Occupational Health Nurses Journal* 46(8): 391–403

Perkins, R., Petrie, K., Alley, P., Barnes, P., Fisher, M. and Hatfield, P. (1997). 'Health service reform: the perceptions of medical specialists in Australia (New South Wales), the United Kingdom and New Zealand', *Medical Journal of Australia* 167: 201–4

Pinto, J.K. (2000). 'Understanding the role of politics in successful project management', *International Journal of Project Management*, 18(2): 85–91

PMI (see Project Management Institute)

Polgar, S. and Thomas, S. (2000). *Introduction to Research in the Health Sciences*, 4th edn, Churchill Livingstone, Edinburgh

Pollitt, C. (1995). 'Justification by works or by faith? Evaluating the new public management', in *Evaluation*, SAGE Publications, Thousand Oaks, CA, Vol 1:2 pp. 133–54

Project Management Institute (2000). *A Guide to the Project Management Body of Knowledge*, PMI, Newtown Square, Pennsylvania

Project Management Institute (2002). *Information Source Guide 2002*, PMI, Newtown Square, Pennsylvania

Roberts, K. and Ludvigsen, C. (1998). *Project Management for Health Care Professionals*, Butterworth Heinemann, Oxford

Rosenau, M.D.J. (1998). *Successful Project Management*, John Wiley & Sons, New York

Rummler, C.A. and Brache, A.P. (1995). *Improving Performance: How to manage the white space on the organisation chart*, Jossey-Bass, San Francisco

Rubin, H.J and Rubin, I. (1992). 'Project management: planning, funding, implementation, and evaluation,' in *Community Organizing and Development*, 2nd edn, Macmillan, New York

Senge, P. (1990). *The Fifth Discipline*, Random House, New York

Smith, G. (1999). 'Project leadership: Why project management alone doesn't work', *Hospital Material Management Quarterly* 21(1): 88–92

Stephenson, T. (1985). *Management: A Political Activity*, Macmillan, Basingstoke

Stretton, A. (1997). 'Foreword', in P. Healy, *Project Management: Getting the job done on time and in budget*, Butterworth Heinemann, Melbourne

Stromsikova, D. and Skackova, D. (2001). *Searching for Excellence in Project Management: Lecture*, Government Office, Central Department for PHARE Contract, Bratislava, Slovakia

Taylor, C.E. and Reinke, W.A. (1988). 'The process, structure and functions of planning', in W.A. Reinke (ed.), *Health Planning for Effective Management*, Oxford University Press, New York

Van Eyk, H., Baum, F. and Houghton, G. (2001). 'Coping with health care reform', *Australian Health Review* 24(2): 202–6

Verzuh, E. (1999). *The Fast Forward MBA in Project Management*, John Wiley & Sons Inc., New York

Wadsworth, Y. (1990). *Everyday Evaluation on the Run*, Action Research Issues Association, Victoria

Walker, R. (2001). 'Trust between primary health care organisations', *Health Promotion Journal of Australia* 11(1): 43–7

Webster, G. (1999). *Managing Projects at Work*, Gower Publishing Ltd, Hampshire, UK

Weiser, M. and Morrison, J. (1998). 'Project memory: Information management for project teams', *Journal of Management Information Systems* 14(4): 149–66

White, D. and Fortune, J. (2002). 'Current practice in project management: An empirical study', *International Journal of Project Management* 20(1): 1–11

Williams, R. (1980). 'Literature and sociology', in R. Williams, *Problems in Materialism and Culture*, Verso, London

Wilson, G. and Wright, M. (1993). *Evaluation Framework*, CDIH, Melbourne

Young, T.L. (1997). *How to be a Better Project Manager*, Kogan Page, London

Zimmer, B. (1999a). 'Project Management: Breakthrough or bust', *Hospital Material Management Quarterly* 21(1): 93–9

Zimmer, B. (1999b). 'Project management: A methodology for success', *Hospital Material Management Quarterly* 21(2): 82–9

Index